Intellectual Disability and Mental Health:

A Training Manual in Dual Diagnosis

Sharon McGilvery, Ph.D.
and
Darlene Sweetland, Ph.D.

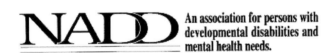
LCCN: 2011941140
ISBN: 978-1-57256-070-3

1st Printing 2011

Printed in the United States of America

Acknowledgements

There are many people who supported us in writing this book. We would like to express our gratitude to Kimberly Gaines-Williams, Ph.D., for her assistance in editing and Kathy Karins, RN, for her expertise in reviewing the medical chapter of the book. We would also like to acknowledge the support provided by Community Services of the San Diego Regional Center, specifically Dan Clark, LCSW.

I would like to thank my following colleagues: Karen Whittler, LCSW, Michael Raulston, LCSW, Lynne Gregory, Ph.D., Ellen O'Neal, RN, and Ray Vagas, Ph.D., for their support throughout the years and their dedication to enriching the lives of individuals with developmental disorders.

I would like to thank my husband, Alden T. Merrill III, for his patience, humor, and for keeping the home fires burning throughout the process of writing this book.

-Sharon McGilvery

I would like to personally thank Peggie Webb of Mosaic Connections who provided not only professional guidance, but support and encouragement throughout this process. In addition, the San Diego Regional Center has been a strong supporter of the Solutions Building Community Collaborative, a demonstration project sponsored by the San Diego Regional Center and San Diego County Mental Health. This is a collaborative effort across multiple systems with a specific focus on adults who are dually served with high frequency, high intensity behaviors that result in the frequent use of crisis services.

I would also like to thank my husband, Ron Stolberg, for not only his patience and support, but his technological skill and reviewer's eye.

-Darlene Sweetland

Table of Contents

Introduction

Throughout our years of working in the field of intellectual disability, we have had the privilege of sharing our experience and knowledge with a variety of people from medical and mental health professionals to teachers and law enforcement personnel. Our audiences have also included direct care staff and families. By providing trainings and consultations to people with diverse backgrounds, we have been able to identify the areas that provide some of the greatest concerns and generate the most questions.

As a result of inquiries from audiences and their desire to learn more about how to serve individuals with an intellectual disability and psychiatric conditions, this book was written. This book is primarily designed for direct care providers, such as social workers, counselors, and direct care staff. However, it is hoped that some of the information may be useful as either reminders to those already knowledgeable in this area or as areas for further reflection among skilled clinicians. The goal of this book is to provide practical guidelines and tools that can be used immediately. It is also intended to provide guidelines on how to ensure more comprehensive care for this population, whether or not you are the provider of clinical services or the provider of day-to-day care. Consequently, its content spans the gamut from assessment to intervention. For those who wish to learn more, including detailed research findings and theory beyond the scope of this manuscript, there are great books available. Two such books are: *Dual Diagnosis: An Introduction to the Mental Health Needs of Person with Developmental Disabilities* by Griffiths, Stavrakaki, and Summers (2002) and *Diagnostic Manual-Intellectual Disability: A Textbook of Diagnosis of Mental Disorders in Persons with Intellectual Disability* (Fletcher, Loschen, Stavrakaki, & First, 2007b).

This book was designed to help bridge the gap between the mental health system and the developmental disabilities system and further enhance services to individuals who are dually diagnosed (having co-occurring intellectual disability and mental illness). This book addresses assessment, treatment, and training. It also addresses complicating factors in identifying appropriate psychiatric diagnoses for individuals with developmental disorders, as well as the significant underreporting of psychiatric disorders for this population. It includes new ways of looking at assessment and treatment, such as intervention strategies and treatment accommodations, when working with individuals with developmental disorders. It is hoped that in the content of this book we have communicated our respect and empathy for the challenges they face and the many lessons they teach.

The term *developmental disabilities* encompasses a number of disorders including intellectual disabilities, autism spectrum disorders, genetic disorders, sensory-related disorders, and degenerative disorders. This book was written to discuss the complicating factors of working with individuals with an *intellectual disability;* however, much of the information provided is relevant for individuals with other developmental disabilities as well.

In appreciating the opportunities provided by working with this population, I am reminded of a documentary I saw on television. It was a documentary about a Canadian Indian tribe in which a non-tribal psychologist, using a battery of psychological tests, assessed a child. The results indicated that she had an intellectual disability within the severe range. The psychologist was sympathetic and almost apologetic to the family's plight. The family responded with a great deal of concern. A psychologist who was a member of the tribe intervened due to the family's level of distress. However, instead of being sympathetic he congratulated the family, and the family's distress turned to appreciation and joy. When the first psychologist witnessed this, he was alarmed and asked why the family was congratulated. The tribal psychologist stated that in their culture if a family had a child with an intellectual disability they were considered to be privileged. It was their tribe's spiritual belief that the child was placed on Earth to help develop the human skills of compassion, wisdom, and patience. Therefore, any family privileged to have such a teacher among them was to be congratulated. It is in this spirit that this book was written. The lessons learned from working with individuals with an intellectual disability have been invaluable on many levels. They continue to serve as our teachers, and it is their instructions and voices that have provided the lessons presented in this book.

Chapter 1

Dual Diagnoses:
The Scope of the Challenge

Working with people who have both an intellectual disability and psychiatric illnesses provides many challenges, as well as rewards. This field has been evolving, and there is now a greater understanding of the fact that psychiatric conditions not only occur among this population but that they may occur with greater frequency (Reiss, 1990). At one time, it was assumed that a person with an intellectual disability could not have a psychiatric disorder. Behavioral challenges were viewed as either learned behavior or behaviors attributed to the intellectual disability. Over time, the possibility that psychiatric disorders could exist for individuals with an intellectual disability became generally accepted.

The lives of individuals with both intellectual disabilities and psychiatric conditions can be complex and challenging. The level of supports and services needed to assist individuals with dual diagnoses requires a heightened awareness of their unique needs. It requires a special sensitivity to all challenges they may encounter.

Diagnostic Considerations

Being aware of the diagnostic challenges that exist in serving this population is critical. The signs and symptoms of certain psychiatric disorders often present in atypical or unusual ways. These can be the result of limitations in language and cognitive abilities, as well as limitations in life experiences and opportunities. Because the symptom presentation is often atypical, symptoms can be misinterpreted by others as being purely behavioral. For example, it is not uncommon for behavioral responses to be classified as attention-seeking, willful, or resistive. Individuals may develop negative reputations because of long histories of significant behavioral challenges. It is important to be more aware that these responses may be psychiatric in origin.

Among the general population, the diagnosis of a psychiatric condition is based largely on symptom self-report, the results of mental status examinations, clinical observations, standardized testing, and other collateral information obtained by the clinician. For individuals with intellectual disabilities, the use of these traditional information gathering sources is often hindered by cognitive limitations and expressive language skill deficits. In individuals who are cognitively functioning within the profound and severe range of intellectual disabilities, expressive language skills are frequently absent or severely limited. In addition, the limited life experiences and personal resources of individuals who are dually diagnosed tend to alter the more typical presentation of psychiatric symptoms. For example, an individual diagnosed with bipolar disorder in the general population may acquire financial debt in a manic phase. An individual with an intellectual disability who lives in an institution has neither the financial resources nor opportunity to incur financial debt. Therefore, the atypical presentation of psychiatric illnesses for individuals who are dually diagnosed presents a diagnostic challenge. It may result in questions of reliability and validity of the diagnostic process and the diagnosis itself.

Obtaining an accurate diagnosis can be a time-consuming process. It takes time to ensure possible medical issues are ruled out as causes of, or contributors to, the diagnosis. Often, histories of symptoms may be missing due to residential changes. The individual may have moved many times, resulting in changes of care providers. The coordination of care among medical professionals can also be a time-consuming task. Finally, the diagnostic process can be further hindered when the individual's symptoms are attributed to the intellectual disability rather than to a specific psychiatric disorder.

System Challenges

It can be a challenge to identify and obtain the appropriate psychiatric and psychological services to address the psychiatric disorders. There is a shortage of medical providers who have both the background and interest in working with this population. In addition, it is sometimes difficult to access those resources, even when available, because of the individual's own resistance to medical care. Individuals with an intellectual disability, particularly those who are cognitively functioning within the severe and profound range, may be fearful and resist medical and psychiatric care. They may refuse to get out of vehicles or leave the physicians' offices before the appointments are completed. They may feel uncomfortable about being examined, and subsequently avoid being touched. Such resistiveness can delay a diagnosis and treatment.

Even when appropriate medical and psychiatric services are obtained, there may be disruptions in the continuity of care based on psychiatric hospitalizations and changes in living arrangements. For example, if the behavioral challenges necessitate a periodic admission to a psychiatric hospital, it is often the case that the inpatient psychiatrist is not the outpatient treating psychiatrist. This can lead to numerous medication changes with an increased potential for side effects. In addition, a behavioral crisis may result in an emergency discharge notice from the individual's group home. Consequently, upon discharge from the psychiatric hospital, the individual will now have a new home to go to and a new treating psychiatrist. The records may or may not follow the individual after the move. This can further complicate and hinder care. Changes in residences can also lead to changes in neurologists, physicians, psychologists, etc. The medical providers are sometimes tasked to start from the beginning, which can lead to delays in treatment. In addition, the medical diagnostic process can be time-consuming, and the financial compensation can be less than the medical providers would normally receive.

Transient placements can also cause problems. Sometimes when emergency placements are required, the person is placed in a residence that does not have the appropriate resources. An emergency placement may occur for several reasons. It may occur out of necessity if the person no longer meets criteria for continued admission to a psychiatric hospital or it may occur if the person's home issued a discharge notice. This leaves little time to identify an appropriate resource when the change occurs.

If the individual has to change residences, this will often mean the person's job or day program changes. Consequently, every area of the person's life may be undergoing change. This could add to further instability in the person's life and result in greater stress.

The systems which support individuals with dual diagnoses can themselves be in a state of flux. Budgetary restraints and changes can result in the termination or reduction of services. They may leave the person with decreased access to medical, psychiatric, psychological, and even recreational services. Consequently, negotiating the systems, along with negotiating the daily stressors and challenges, can be a daunting task.

Daily Stressors

The daily stressors experienced by this population can contribute to psychiatric disorders, and in some situations even create them. It is not unusual for an individual with a dual diagnosis to have an extensive residential history. This can contribute to fears and concerns about rejection, abandonment, and anxiety in general. For individuals who are cognitively functioning within the mild to moderate range of an intellectual disability, numerous discharges from facilities or homes can add to a sense of self-defeat, low self-esteem, and fear of making another mistake. Care providers may experience burn-out as a result of dealing with the behavioral challenges. Families may be estranged because they have grown weary of the individual's mental health issues and behavioral challenges. Frequent discharge notices or out-of-home placements can contribute to loss issues and further disruptions in attachment histories. Upon being discharged from a facility, there may be little or no time to say good-bye to the people the person has come to trust or rely upon. These factors can lead to a history of instability in interpersonal relationships, living arrangements, and social support networks.

Adding to the interpersonal stressors, there can be a high rate of staff change in many facilities. Individuals with dual diagnoses may find themselves having to adjust to numerous staffing changes and a variety of different personalities among their care providers. Sometimes care providers may expect too little from the individuals they support. They may perform daily tasks that the person is able to do or is capable of learning. Consequently, this interferes with the person's ability to develop self-confidence and become more independent.

To add to the challenges already posed, there is also the increased possibility of abuse among this population. If the person experienced abuse in the past, it could increase the likelihood of posttraumatic stress reactions and symptoms of anxiety later. Sometimes, the individual is not able to articulate that he or she has been the victim of abuse by a care provider. However, the person's behaviors may be symptomatic of traumatic reactions including an increased level of arousal or fear. Limited verbal and cognitive skills may render the individual helpless to disclose the abuse history and the impact those experiences have on day-to-day functioning and stress levels. In addition, the individual's reliance on care providers may result in a reluctance to do or say anything that may anger the person who is caring for him or her.

A Future Commitment

What has become evident over the past few decades is the ever increasing need to expand our knowledge about intellectual disability and psychiatric disorders. With the increased identification of psychiatric disorders among this population, it is important to ensure that care providers and medical personnel are educated about the supports and services needed.

The benefits of increasing knowledge in this area are numerous. It not only improves the quality of the lives of the people we work with and their families, but it also has an added benefit for professionals and care providers. Individuals with an intellectual disability have not received the appreciation or recognition that is due in a society that values intellectual abilities. Ironically, the lessons that this population can contribute to care providers and clinicians can be invaluable. Working with this population can highlight the importance of "going back to basics." For example, the basic diagnostic hierarchy for a mental health clinician is to rule out any medical causes of the symptoms first. All of the psychiatric diagnoses in the current *Diagnostic and Statistical Manual of Mental Disorders-Fourth Edition-Text Revision* (American Psychiatric Association, 2000), have a qualifier which states that medical causes should be excluded before rendering a psychiatric diagnosis. For individuals with an intellectual disability, particularly those individuals who lack the expressive language skills, it is imperative to rule out any underlying medical causes of behavioral challenges or psychiatric symptoms. This type of thoroughness and attention to detail can only help clinicians in their general practice. It can help prevent an error in diagnosis and improper treatment. Working with individuals with dual diagnoses also emphasizes the need to coordinate care among treating professionals. This type of approach benefits everyone. It benefits practitioners who serve the general population as well as those who serve this special population.

Working with this population also provides some refreshing perspectives. For example, sometimes there is a purity of thought which is novel to encounter. You may not have to meander through fields of psychological defense mechanisms such as rationalizations or intellectualizations. People with an intellectual disability may "call it like they see it" and wear their hearts on their sleeves. I am reminded of my first introduction to someone with an intellectual disability. It was my neighbor's son who was 7 years-old and had Down syndrome. He was riding his tricycle up our brick pathway one day. He hit a misplaced brick and fell off his bike. I ran to help him and asked him if he was alright. He got up, dusted himself off, and answered my question by saying, "Of course I am not all right. I just fell." As a little girl I remember being struck by his honesty and lack of pretense. He wasn't embarrassed. He wasn't ashamed. He was hurt with scrapes and bruises and seemingly surprised and annoyed by my question.

Working with individuals with an intellectual disability has the added benefit of reminding us of the importance of freedom of choice. Among this population, individuals sometimes have few choices in their lives. They may not have been able to choose where they live or who they are going to live with. They may have little or no input into how their days are structured or what day programs or vocational programs they attend. It reminds us of how important it is to be surrounded by activities and people we enjoy and how fortunate we are to have our freedoms. It also reminds us of how the power of choice increases the quality of life. This is an essential part of any support offered to those we are fortunate to work with and learn about.

Chapter 2

Factors Complicating Psychiatric Diagnoses

The Diagnostic and Statistical Manual of Mental Disorders-Fourth Edition-Text Revision (*DSM-IV-TR*, American Psychiatric Association, 2000) is the diagnostic system most commonly used to identify psychiatric conditions. This manual has been revised several times and has included more diagnoses and diagnostic criteria over the years. The *DSM-IV-TR* contains over 300 diagnoses. While it assists clinicians in communicating about the clinical picture of individuals with mental health disorders, the symptoms may look different for people with an intellectual disability.

Individuals with an intellectual disability can experience the same psychiatric disorders as those seen among the general population. In fact, while estimates of the rate of psychiatric disorders among individuals with an intellectual disability have varied, they have generally been quoted as being higher than in the general population. Some studies have reported that approximately 10% to 40% of individuals with intellectual disabilities have a co-existing mental illness (Reiss, 1990). Other studies have presented higher prevalence rates ranging from 30% to 70% (Szymanki & King, 1999). The range in findings can be attributable to a variety of factors including differences in population sampling and difficulties accurately identifying psychiatric disorders among this population.

The term *dual diagnosis* is used when an individual is diagnosed with more than one major disorder. The term *mental illness* as defined by Reiss, Goldberg, and Ryan (1993) is a "Severe disturbance of behavior, mood, thought processes and/or social and interpersonal relationships" (p. 1). Historically, the term dual diagnosis has been used to refer to an individual with a substance abuse diagnosis and a mental illness. However, the term is also used to refer to an individual with an intellectual disability and a psychiatric disorder. The latter definition is the subject of this book.

While psychiatric disorders may be more prevalent for individuals with an intellectual disability, accurately diagnosing the conditions can be difficult. In fact, it is typically a challenging behavior that prompts a care provider to find out what might be happening for the person. If the behavior is addressed without considering an underlying mental health disorder, the interventions are likely to be ineffective. Take the example of a person who presents with repetitive questions and becomes aggressive when the questions are not answered. The behavioral interpretation may be that the individual is attention-seeking and/or manipulative. On the other hand, the emotional interpretation may be that the person is anxious, depressed, or experiencing paranoia. The treatment interventions are very different depending on the cause of the behavioral challenge.

Barriers to Diagnosis and Treatment

There are numerous factors which complicate the accurate identification of a psychiatric diagnosis among individuals with an intellectual disability. Developmentally, medically, and socially, their behavioral profiles can be complex. When identifying an accurate diagnosis several complications must be considered.

1. **Diagnostic overshadowing.** Reiss, Leviton, and Szyszko (1982) developed the term diagnostic overshadowing to indicate the tendency to attribute many of the possible symptoms of a psychiatric disorder to the intellectual disability. For example, when a person with an intellectual disability communicates being upset by acting out, it can be defined as a behavioral challenge. The fact that it could also be a symptom of a psychiatric disorder is often overlooked. The psychiatric diagnosis is overshadowed by the focus on changing the behavior. Missing a psychiatric diagnosis could lead to improper treatment or no treatment at all.

2. **Problems with polypharmacy.** The rate of polypharmacy with this population is significant. These individuals are often on multiple medications, some of which are treating the same thing. Some of the side effects of the medication can produce symptoms that are similar to a psychiatric disorder. For example, fatigue, confusion, agitation,

lethargy, short attention span, or changes in sleep or appetite are common medication side effects. They are also symptoms of mental health disorders.

3. **Communication deficits.** When attempting to understand a person's experience and how to help them, usually there are a lot of questions posed. If the individual's verbal ability or insight is limited, that person is not likely to provide an accurate presentation of symptoms. For individuals with a profound and severe intellectual disability, the diagnoses need to rely heavily on observable behavioral symptoms and reports from care providers.

4. **Atypical presentation of psychiatric disorders.** It is not uncommon for psychiatric disorders to present as problematic behaviors among individuals with intellectual disabilities. For example, a person with an intellectual disability may not typically express depression by sleeping a lot or having low energy. Instead, depression may be expressed by the individual acting agitated, being easily angered, or engaging in increasingly unsafe behaviors. The focus then becomes managing the behavior rather than exploring whether or not the behavior is a manifestation of an undiagnosed psychiatric condition. In addition, in some instances the behaviors exhibited do not quite meet the accepted threshold of criteria for *DSM-IV-TR*. In which case, the crucial question becomes, "Are the symptoms close enough to meet the diagnostic criteria for a particular disorder?"

5. **Limited life experiences.** Due to a narrow range of life experiences, it may be difficult to detect some of the symptoms of a psychiatric disorder. For example, a typically developing individual with bipolar disorder who is in a manic phase may spend excessively and charge up credit cards or increase social activity, sometimes to an unsafe level. An individual with an intellectual disability may not have the opportunity to have the financial resources for overspending, promiscuous relationships, travel, etc. Therefore, the diagnosis may be missed because the symptoms look different.

6. **Complications of untreated medical conditions.** Untreated medical conditions can present as psychiatric symptoms. For example, some heart conditions can cause symptoms of anxiety. This is further complicated by the fact that some individuals with intellectual disability may not be compliant with medical evaluations and procedures. Care providers are not trained to assess medical conditions, and they, therefore, are less likely to consider consulting with a medical doctor if it means it will upset the individual. For this

reason, medical evaluations may not be scheduled or completed. There is also a shortage of medical providers who want to serve individuals with an intellectual disability. Consequently, finding prompt and comprehensive medical care may be compromised at times.

7. **Acquiescence.** Interviewing someone who has an intellectual disability and obtaining accurate information about the individual's symptoms can be confounded by an increased tendency for the person to agree quickly. The person may tell the clinician or care provider what he or she thinks the interviewer wants to hear or agree to things in order to avoid the risk of disapproval. The person may be more likely to report "yes" or "no" to all questions despite the true response. The interview can also be compromised if the individual has a short attention span and has difficulty attending to the content of the question. Quick answers may be provided in order to shorten the length of the interview.

8. **Imitative or learned behavior.** The individual may be exhibiting behaviors that have been modeled by others. For example, a person may talk about suicide or hearing voices following a psychiatric hospitalization where other people were heard talking about the subject. The person may imitate these behaviors because it was observed that others received attention for doing so.

9. **Lack of behavioral challenges.** If a person is withdrawn or passive, a psychiatric condition (as well as a medical condition) is more likely to be overlooked. Since there are no behavior problems, the individual may be viewed by a care provider as not having any difficulties, when, in fact, the withdrawal or change in functioning may be an indication of a depression or other psychiatric condition. Sometimes a change in the individual's functioning or skill level may be interpreted as improvement if behavior problems are no longer being exhibited. This may actually be a decrease in functioning.

10. **Sensory impairments.** It is important to consider whether the individual has any sensory impairments (sight, hearing, touch, etc.). For example, it is not usual for an individual who is totally blind to have disruptions in sleep. Therefore, diagnosing depression based on changes in sleep as one criterion, or diagnosing a sleep disorder in light of these disruptions, may be inaccurate. Similarly, it is not unusual for a person with a hearing impairment to become agitated with changes in a schedule because not having heard the conversations about making new plans, the person finds the changes expected.

Emotional and Cognitive Considerations

When working with individuals with the complicated profiles of intellectual disabilities and co-existing psychiatric disorders, there are many things to consider. Among those are the emotional and cognitive factors that are unique to this population. The following section includes things to consider when assessing the individual, as well as guidelines to address some of the complications.

Emotional considerations. When working with individuals diagnosed with intellectual disabilities it is important to remember they are progressing through typical developmental milestones, but at a slower pace. Because of this, they are often treated as much younger than their age. Their caregivers may feel that because of their intellectual disabilities they cannot do things for themselves. Tasks are more often completed for them, and choices are often made for them. Because of these challenges, an individual who is progressing through typical developmental stages at a slower pace is now an individual who is having typical developmental desires but little opportunity to experience and learn from the new challenges.

Adults with mild and high moderate levels of intellectual disabilities are likely to be going through the following developmental changes:

- Desire for increased independence
- Desire to make their own choices
- Desire for more long-term relationships
- Feeling confused with the new challenges and responsibilities

If the person also has a psychiatric disorder, chances are he or she is in an environment with even more supervision and less opportunity to meet these developmental desires. This can cause a lot of frustration and confusion. With each transitional stage or developmental shift, there is the likelihood that it will be accompanied by an increase in problem behavior, difficulties adjusting to changes, and variable emotional states. Just as with the general population, this is normal. It can also be a time of excitement and pride at the new skills which can be mastered.

A question that is very often asked is "How do you treat an individual as an adult when the person presents as child-like?" To address this it may be helpful to follow this guideline:

*Offer an environment that offers **age appropriate opportunities** (job, home, relationships, self-help responsibilities), while providing **developmentally appropriate supports** (supervision, coaching, education).*

Relationships. Relationship problems are a common cause for a person with a dual diagnosis to be referred to a behavior consultant. This can include relationships with parents, peers, bosses, romantic interests, caregivers, and strangers. It is a challenge to provide a person with an intellectual disability *and* a co-existing psychiatric disorder typical experiences in regards to relationships. Often it is difficult for these individuals to live safely at home; therefore, they are in out-of-home placements. Their residential histories may be extensive, making it less likely for them to have formed peer relationships. The people they most often interact with are "staff;" therefore their experiences developing healthy relationships are limited.

In addition, because of their life circumstances (group homes, day programs, limited social interactions), individuals with dual diagnoses often do not have the opportunity to explore romantic relationships in a healthy way. For many adults with an intellectual disability romantic relationships are often discouraged. Consequently, they don't have the opportunity to learn about how to have a relationship with a partner and establish appropriate boundaries.

Some patterns that result from these atypical experiences are a misunderstanding about boundaries in relationships. You may see them become very strict with boundaries and not expect anyone to stay in their life or really support them. Conversely, you may see the opposite pattern, where they become overly close to others whom they do not know well. Recently, with the increase in technological communication, there has been the added risk of meeting people on-line. This can be very confusing for people who have not learned about healthy boundaries in relationships. They may believe what people are telling them, be eager to make friends, and schedule meetings. This can be potentially dangerous.

Adults with an intellectual disability often have the developmental desires of adolescents. However, while pre-teens and adolescents are given additional responsibility and independence to develop and mature, individuals with an intellectual disability are often protected. They are not thought to be capable and are consequently limited in their relational experiences. This is not only frustrating for that person, but they miss the experience necessary to make mistakes and learn from them. Addressing this need and providing education and opportunities for healthy adult relationships are very important.

Alternately, if individuals have not had the experiences of developing positive long-term attachments to others, they may be less likely to attend to other people's feelings and reactions. This is not because they are uncaring, but because they never learned they matter in relationships. For example, care providers may find themselves wondering why the people they support continue to curse and call them names when it means they are not able to participate in outings. Individuals with an intellectual disability who do not understand the role their behaviors play in interpersonal interactions may not make the connection between calling people names and people not wanting to spend time with them.

The best way to provide experiences that are positive in regards to relationships is to understand a person's relational history. It is important to recognize the individual's experiences with relationships and understand what the person has learned to expect from them. For example, did the person have the opportunity to form attachments with early parental figures, whether they were biological parents, relatives, or foster parents? What is the longest time the person has known someone and had that individual involved in his or her life? Additional factors to consider are:

1. *What is the person's family involvement?*
   a. How long did the person live at home as a child?
   b. Does the person still have family relationships?
   c. How often does the individual see family members and are the visits positive?
   d. Are extended family members involved?

2. *What is the person's living arrangement?*
   a. How long has the person lived in the current home?
   b. How frequently has the person moved or have living arrangements been stable?
   c. What is the individual's history of out-of-home placements?
   d. What were the staffing patterns in the past homes (staff run, owner occupied, etc.)?

3. *Is there a history of abuse?*
   a. How long ago was the abuse?
   b. What was the relationship with the person?
   c. Was the abuse reported and what was the outcome?

4. *Who are the individuals who the person has formed attachments with and are they still involved?*
    a. What is the most stable relationship in the person's life?
    b. Is the relationship mutual?
    c. Does the person have peer relationships?
    d. What type of relationships does the person talk about or desire?

5. *What is the person's level of independence in the community?*
    a. Does the person have the skills to form healthy relationships independently?
    b. Does the individual have support from community members (e.g., the employee at the neighborhood coffee shop, etc.)?

6. *What is the individual's work history?*
    a. What was the person's highest level of functioning?
    b. Does the individual have peer interactions at work? Are those interactions desired?
    c. Does the person interact with others regularly at work?

The interventions and supports are going to differ depending on the answers to these questions. Some people with dual diagnoses have transient residential experiences with minimal family involvement. That means, of the people they currently have contact with, the longest relationship may be a year or less. This experience will have a considerable impact on their current relationships and how they treat others.

Cognitive considerations. Any time a diagnosis, behavior strategy, or intervention is considered, the cognitive profile of the individual needs to be evaluated. By definition, a person with an intellectual disability has a disorder in cognitive functioning. The specific function of the disorder differs for each person. At the same time there are some processes that are common. This section includes some guidelines about improving our ability to communicate so our message is more easily understood and remembered. Cognitive processes that are often compromised include: receptive and expressive language, short-term memory, long-term retrieval, and executive functioning. The next section will include the cognitive processes that are compromised and guidelines about how to accommodate for these compromised processes.

Expressive Language. A person with poor expressive language is likely to have a lot of difficulty expressing thoughts and ideas verbally. Just as with the general population, this will be even more difficult if the person is emotionally overwhelmed. The individual may complain about others, make a lot of requests to staff, or want attention from staff, as a means to communicate feelings. The person may also use unsafe or "attention getting" behaviors to let others know that staff support is needed. Often an individual with an intellectual disability will use behavior to communicate instead of words. *Behavioral expressions* are non-verbal ways for a person to communicate what he or she is thinking and/or feeling. Most often *behavioral expressions* are complex or multiple non-verbal acts used to communicate. For example, a person may begin to pace, then yell, and then throw a chair as a way to communicate feelings of anxiety. The individual is not using verbal expressions to communicate feelings, but instead is using behaviors. Behavioral expressions and brief verbal communications are just as important in understanding a person as a lengthy dialogue.

Guidelines
1. Be a good listener.
2. Summarize what message you heard from the person. This lets the person know you understand, and it helps to consolidate the message.
3. Be patient. It may take some time for the individual to express his or her concern.
4. Don't try to answer for the person, if possible. The person may be agreeing for approval or to end the conversation. The agreement may not be what the person is feeling.
5. Don't get caught up in the accuracy of all of the details; instead focus on the feeling. Often the details will be inaccurate, but it is not related to what the person is trying to communicate. Correcting all of the details can frustrate the person and lead the conversation off the original point.
6. Be very attentive to *behavioral expressions.* Behavioral expressions are just as important as verbal expressions.

Receptive language. A person with poor receptive language can become easily overwhelmed with too much verbal input or instruction. Abstract words and terms are generally not understood or remembered. This is important because so much of our communication is verbal. It is a natural tendency to want to "explain" something as a teaching tool. Explaining is very valuable, however, it is important to monitor the amount of information that is communicated verbally. Individuals with poor receptive language can become overwhelmed with the amount of information and then not remember any of it.

Guidelines

1. Decide on your message and the point of your discussion. Stick to that point.
2. Focus on one goal at a time. Don't include other, albeit equally important, "lessons" in the discussion. Save them for another discussion where you focus on only one of those lessons.
3. Use the person's frame of reference to provide examples. This way the person is not always learning new material.
4. Don't use abstract words or terms. For example, instead of saying "That was not appropriate", say "That was not nice" or "That made him want to move away from you."
5. Be a good listener. The individual may be processing what you are saying by talking about the ideas out loud.
6. Provide visual cues and examples whenever possible. Drawings and charts of what you are discussing can be great tools. As you are discussing the person's goals, you can draw a line with where the individual is now and what the expectations are as the final goal is reached.
7. Encourage them to keep a notebook that includes important information. They can make notes or drawings or can ask someone to do that for them.

Short-term memory. Memory is often significantly impacted for individuals with an intellectual disability. This occurs because of the neurological factors of their disabilities as well as side effects of some of the medications. Because memory is commonly impaired anyway, medication side effects such as fatigue, loss of concentration, or increased agitation can impair memory even further. This is especially true for short-term memory.

Short-term memory is required when you need to maintain formation in memory for a very short period of time. For example, u are trying to remember a phone number and you need to it over and over until you write it down, that is using your short-mory. Once you are distracted or you think about something rget it. It is forgotten because it was never integrated m memory. Individuals with an intellectual disability hort attention spans and more trouble focusing for long-periods of time. Individuals with dual diagnoses are often emotionally overwhelmed and easily distracted. This makes them even more vulnerable to distractions in highly emotional situations. This is very important to remember because if instructions are given during this time, they may have a lot of difficulty remembering them. For example, if someone is feeling anxious and the doctor is talking about medications, the person is likely to forget the instructions.

Guidelines

1. Assess a person's emotional state before providing a lot of new information.
2. Provide any instructions in writing (or pictures).
3. Check in with the person a few minutes after the information is given to assess how much of it was remembered.
4. Always be patient and supportive when instructions need to be repeated.
5. Communicate with the person in a quiet environment with minimal distractions.

Long-term retrieval. One of the most common challenges for people with an intellectual disability is retrieving information from long-term memory. This means that they have the information stored in their long-term memory; they just have difficulty recalling and communicating it. Therefore, open-ended questions are more difficult to answer. When presented with an open-ended question they will often provide the same response or one of only a few responses. This is as true for an everyday question, "What do you want for dinner?", as it is for an emotionally focused question such as, "What can you do to help yourself calm down?" You will find that often these individuals will resort to past patterns of coping and behavioral reactions when they are overwhelmed. This makes sense because it is very difficult to come up with different options. For example, someone who is depressed may frequently ask to go to the hospital because that is the individual's regular response to feeling depressed.

Guidelines

1. Avoid open-ended questions when possible. Open-ended questions require an individual to identify multiple options from which to choose, such as, "What do you want to do today?" or "Why did you do that?"
2. Follow-up an open-ended question with some possible options. These options can be presented verbally or, better

yet, in picture form (or a written list).

3. When new options are identified, add them to a list for the person to refer to for future reference.

4. Use picture lists of options as a way to provide choices. This is great for people who are verbally fluent as well as non-verbal. It takes away the factor of retrieval when making a choice. If the list is in written form (pictures or words), the options can be endless. For example, a list of coping skills is a great tool so when they are most overwhelmed they are not dependent on long-term retrieval.

5. Refer to past information or written plans as a reference.

Executive functioning. Executive functioning refers to multi-step processes such as planning, organizing, initiating, concentrating, problem-solving, and multi-tasking. Consider how many people organize their day. They think about what time they need to leave to get to work on time and plan what tasks they need to complete, dealing with unexpected changes in their schedule, running errands on their break, planning around the schedules of family members, completing household chores, etc. Most people do this every day and don't think about all that goes into organizing these tasks. They are using executive functioning.

Executive functioning is something that is very difficult for individuals with an intellectual disability and something that staff and care providers often take for granted. It is more apparent when considering how it relates to a person's ability to organize something concrete such as a schedule or self-help skill (cooking, laundry). For example, when preparing a meal a person needs to plan the ingredients, timing, materials, recipe, and food preparation. That is all needed to complete the single task. Now think about how executive functioning can be compromised when a person is expected to use good judgment when agitated, angry, depressed, or anxious. Not only is the person expected to access "good coping skills," but the person is expected to do so despite being distracted by the emotionally charged situation. Executive functioning is needed in emotional situations as much, if not more, than in routine situations. When identifying supports, teaching skills, and designing behavior plans it is important to consider how to teach coping skills that decrease or executive functioning.

Guidelines as they relate to routines:

1. Written plans can be the best references for an individual. The person can always refer to them without relying on executive functioning.
2. Any written plan should be a working document that is added to and revised as the person has new thoughts and ideas.
3. When making a request, make sure it is close to the time you would like the task completed.
4. Routines are very important to help a person remain independent without having to rely on executive functioning.
5. Help the person solve problems one step at a time. Work consecutively and avoid language that can be confusing, such as "if."
6. Break down daily hygiene tasks into individual steps. Each step can be paired with a picture cue.

Guidelines as they relate to coping skills:

1. Develop a picture chart that represents all of the things the person finds calming (music, exercise, deep breathing, cooking, walking, bath, etc.).
2. Develop an automatic response to have the person calm his or her body before solving the problem. This can be done by saying "Let's calm your body before I help you solve the problem."
3. Don't get caught up in the details of the problem when the person is agitated, but focus on helping the individual become physically calm and understand the frustration.
4. Unstructured time makes a person with a dual diagnosis more vulnerable to increasing anxiety. Therefore, provide a structured schedule of activities. Included in the activity options can be "relax" or "listen to music." Sometimes having an activity board or card that is individualized to the particular person is helpful. The board or card should only include activities that are available to the person at the time. For example, if going to a movie is not a viable option, it should not be offered as a choice.

This is a group of people who tend to require a lot of time on the part of the support team. Determining accurate diagnoses and correct treatment interventions can be a complicated and overwhelming process. At the same time, if these are not considered, more time is likely to be spent later if diagnoses are missed or inaccurate. This summary of guidelines can serve as a simple reminder so that each area is considered:

First: Discuss as a team **all of the possible reasons** for the person's challenges. Make sure that medical and psychological supports are used to rule in, rule out, or defer each possible reason.

Second: Consider the person's **developmental level** and goals and achievements appropriate to that person's developmental needs.

Third: Consider the person's **emotional development** and how the person's experiences and history may impact current relationships and awareness of how the individual's interactions are impacting others.

Fourth: Make sure **accommodations** are made to reduce the emphasis on using cognitive processes that are inherently difficult.

Chapter 3

Atypical Presentation of Specific Psychiatric Diagnoses

Individuals with an intellectual disability may have any of the mental health disorders that occur in the general population. Because the symptom presentations are often different, they can be missed. The focus of this section will be on mental health disorders that are commonly seen with people with dual diagnoses. Included are additional considerations when utilizing the diagnostic criteria stated in the *Diagnostic Statistical Manual of Mental Disorders-Fourth Edition-Text Revision* (American Psychiatric Association, 2000). These considerations will be descriptive and are intended to provide guidelines for care providers. Another informative source for assessing how psychiatric disorders may appear differently for this population is the *Diagnostic Manual-Intellectual Disability: A Textbook of Diagnosis of Mental Disorders in Persons with Intellectual Disability (DM-ID)*, edited by Fletcher, Loschen, Stavrakaki, and First (2007b). The *DM-ID* was developed to address the limitations of using the *DSM-IV-TR* as a diagnostic manual for individuals with intellectual disabilities. It includes adaptations made to many of the clinical criteria for this population. It is a comprehensive source that provides research resources as well as addresses each of the specific criteria from the *DSM-IV-TR*.

Using *DSM-IV-TR* criteria to accurately diagnose mental health disorders for people with an intellectual disability is challenging in many ways. First, some of the language in the *DSM-IV-TR* is general and confusing. It uses words such as "significant" and "abnormally," which leaves room for differing opinions. For example, for a manic episode it states, "During the period of mood disturbance, three (or more) of the following symptoms have persisted (four if the mood is only irritable) and have been present to a significant degree." Differentiating the behavioral characteristics of a psychiatric disorder from those of an intellectual disability is already difficult. Vague language like this makes it even more complicated.

Second, many psychiatric disorders are enhanced, expressed, and coped with using cognitive processes. Individuals with intellectual disabilities process information differently. While many people internalize thoughts about their disorder and experience, individuals with an intellectual disability typically externalize their experience. They are also going to use more primitive emotional defenses and are often more "raw" in their experiences. For example, a developmentally typical person may be introspective and thoughtful about feeling depressed. This is one reason low motivation, hopelessness, and wanting to stay in bed are common symptoms. A person with an intellectual disability is more likely to be angry at others, impulsive, and agitated in his or her experience of depression. This is one reason acting out, yelling, and low frustration tolerance are common symptoms.

Third, a developmentally typical person is more likely to have responsibilities to consider with work, family and social networks. These increased responsibilities offer the possibility of loss if his or her responsibilities are neglected. A person can lose a job, cause family conflict, or lose friends if responsibilities are not maintained. In addition, focus on fulfilling responsibilities can offer a distraction. A person with an intellectual disability is more likely to have support people to help with responsibilities. Therefore, the motivation and distraction are not there. In addition, the person is less likely to get into unsafe situations (substance abuse, promiscuity, theft, etc.) because of those same external supports.

The following are some of the major diagnostic categories of the *DSM-IV-TR*. These are accompanied by descriptions of the possible variations in the symptom presentation which can occur among individuals with an intellectual disability. This manual is not intended to be a diagnostic manual; therefore, specific diagnostic criteria, such as the number of symptoms required for a diagnosis, will not be included. Because the *DSM-IV-TR* denotes the specific diagnostic criteria for each disorder, it is not needed here. Also, not every diagnosis is discussed. The intention of this chapter is for the reader to have a better understanding of how to consider a psychiatric diagnosis for an individual with an intellectual disability. The purpose of this chapter is to provide information on the most common clinical diagnoses for this population and to describe how they may appear differently for people with an intellectual disability. It is also recommended that the *DM-ID* (Fletcher et al., 2007a, 2007b) be consulted for adaptations of each of the specific *DSM-IV-TR* criteria. For the purposes of this book, it will be assumed that the symptoms are causing significant distress in occupational, social, or other important areas of functioning, are not the result of a medical condition, and, unless noted, are not due to the effects of a substance. The specific characteristics reported that describe a typical presentation of each diagnosis were taken from the *DSM-IV-TR*.

Mood Disorders

Major Depression. The *DSM-IV-TR* criteria include symptoms of depressed mood most of the day, nearly every day, markedly diminished interest or pleasure in almost all activities, significant weight loss when not dieting or weight gain (e.g. a change of more than 5%), insomnia or hypersomnia nearly every day, psychomotor agitation or retardation nearly every day, fatigue or loss of energy nearly every day, feelings of worthlessness or excessive/inappropriate guilt nearly every day, diminished ability to think or concentrate or indecisiveness nearly every day, and recurrent thoughts of death, suicidal ideation (thoughts), or a specific plan for suicide. In addition, at least one of the symptoms must consist of anhedonia (loss of pleasure and interest in activities) or depressed mood.

Dysthymia. In order to meet the criteria for a diagnosis of Dysthymia according to *DSM-IV-TR*, depressed mood must be present for most of the day, for more days than not, as indicated either by self-report or observation by others, for at least two years (children one year). In addition, the symptoms are similar to those of Major Depression. The difference between the two disorders is that Dysthymia is a long-term depression (at least two years) and the severity of the symptoms may be less. A Major Depressive Episode cannot have been present for the first two years of the disturbance.

Individuals with an *intellectual disability and depression* may present with atypical signs. The mood presentation may be one of irritability, as opposed to a classic depressed mood. Many people who feel depressed are introspective in their experience of depression. They brood or think about things that are negative. They also may try to mask the symptoms as a defense against others knowing how they are feeling. This is not typical for a person with an intellectual disability. Individuals with an intellectual disability often do not use cognitive processes to cope. Therefore, they are more expressive with their negative feelings. Individuals with intellectual disabilities are more likely to become agitated easily, exhibit less patience, have an increase in energy (usually manifested as anger), and reject people with whom they have been close. They may become aggressive due to increased irritability. With some individuals there may also be an increase in neediness and attention-seeking behaviors.

Individuals with an intellectual disability may also complain about vague somatic symptoms. They may talk about not feeling well, being "sick," needing the doctor, etc. There may also be a deterioration in cognitive functioning. This could include a rapid intensification of confusion or a decrease in concentration and focus when attending to everyday tasks.

Individuals with an intellectual disability often exhibit the typical neurovegetative signs of depression, regardless of their level of cognitive impairment. Neurovegetative signs include changes in weight, sleep, and energy level. It is particularly important to look for current changes in appetite, as well as a history of any significant weight fluctuations (which could signal previous episodes of depression). Among individuals within the profound and severe ranges of cognitive impairment, a refusal to eat or decreased appetite is often a common symptom. In addition, there is typically a marked decreased interest in activities they usually found enjoyable. They may also be less responsive to reinforcers that are used as part of a behavioral approach (i.e., decreased reinforcer sensitivity). Regression in skills of daily living can also be symptomatic of a depressive disorder, such as the onset of urinary incontinence in an individual who was previously continent. Therefore, a thorough review of records (both current and historical), along with information from care providers, can be essential in evaluating for the presence of depression and identifying a pattern of skill regression, etc.

In assessing for depression, expressions of suicidal ideation and suicidal intent (gestures) may be present but misunderstood and mislabeled. For example, the individual may say, "I want to leave here." This can be misconstrued as a desire to change residences, when, in fact, it may be a statement reflecting suicidal ideation. Suicidal gestures may be misinterpreted and labeled as self-injurious behaviors. The individual may attempt to swallow sharp objects or cut himself or herself which may be mislabeled as pica or self-injurious behavior.

The following is a list of the typical symptoms indicative of a depressive disorder for individuals without an intellectual disability:

Table 1
Behavioral Characteristics of Depression

Typical Presentation	Presentation Common for a Person With an Intellectual Disability
Sad Mood	Agitated or irritable mood
Low energy and motivation	High energy exhibited with anger and agitation
Poor concentration	Poor concentration and low frustration tolerance
Change in eating habits, eating less or more	Change in eating habits, eating less or more
Change in sleeping habits, sleeping less or more	Change in sleeping habits, with sleeping less more typical than sleeping more
Loss of pleasure in activities	Loss of pleasure in activities
Thoughts of harming self	Actions that harm self, expressed wish to be dead

In people who have an intellectual disability, as with any individual, it is important to identify and treat depression. Symptoms of depression can easily be overlooked in individuals with an intellectual disability, particularly among individuals whose cognitive functioning is within the profound and severe range of an intellectual disability. Unfortunately, if their depressive symptoms lead to greater passivity and social withdrawal, they may be considered by care providers as "easy" to deal with and the diagnosis will be overlooked.

Bipolar Disorder. In order to make the diagnosis of Bipolar Disorder according to *DSM-IV-TR* criteria, an individual needs to experience a manic or hypomanic episode. A manic episode is characterized by a distinct period of abnormally and persistently elevated, expansive, or irritable mood lasting at least one week (or any duration if hospitalization is necessary). The *DSM-IV-TR* criteria include symptoms of inflated self-esteem or grandiosity, decreased need for sleep, more talkative than usual or pressure to keep talking, flight of ideas or subjective experience that thoughts are racing, easily distracted, increase in goal-directed activity or psychomotor agitation, and excessive involvement in pleasurable activities that have a high potential for painful consequences.

A *hypomanic episode* is characterized by a distinct period of persistently elevated, expansive, or irritable mood, lasting at least four days, that is clearly different from the usual mood. The duration of the episode is less than that for a manic episode and the number of symptoms needed to meet the criteria are fewer than that for a manic episode.

Bipolar Disorder includes numerous subtypes including Bipolar I Disorder and Bipolar II Disorder. There is also another category of Bipolar Disorder Not Otherwise Specified (NOS) for disorders with bipolar features that do not meet the criteria for Bipolar I or Bipolar II. The exact designation is made only after a thorough history is taken and it is determined if the current mood is depressed, manic, hypomanic, or mixed.

People who are manic experience moods which can be very changeable. Their moods may change from crying, to irritability, to suddenly laughing, each of which can rapidly change. All three moods may be present within a 24-hour period. This is common for individuals with an intellectual disability as well. While the symptoms are similar for individuals with and without an intellectual disability, the behavioral patterns resulting from these symptoms are not. Behavioral patterns may be different due to differing life experiences, opportunities, expressive language skills, and cognitive abilities. Common patterns of mania in individuals with an intellectual disability include the following:

1. *Grandiosity.* Behavioral patterns such as increased spending habits, promiscuous behavior, developing business plans, increased drug and alcohol use, and job changes are common for people experiencing a manic phase. On the other hand, people with an intellectual disability do not typically have access to these resources. Consequently, their limited life experiences and opportunities may lead to a different presentation of symptoms. For example, they may express grandiosity by presenting themselves as a staff member. Since it is not unusual for them to see the staff as people of power, they may identify with this role when they are in a manic episode. Individuals may make plans to change residences or move out on their own, refuse medication, engage in inappropriate social interactions with peers or staff, or engage in hypersexual behaviors. In *DM-ID,* Charlot et al. (2007) note that grandiosity may be expressed as exaggerated claims of skills or stature. They also note that at the "preoperational cognitive stage of development, fantasy and reality are not distinguished. Claims may represent wishes versus mood congruent delusional beliefs" (p. 173). Therefore, the developmental level of the individual must be considered before his or her claims are considered "delusional" or "grandiose".

2. *Rapid and pressured speech.* Individuals in manic states can present with pressured and rapid speech. They may speak rapidly about ideas, plans, and affection for others. However, this may be difficult to detect in people who lack the expressive language skills to communicate such thoughts. In an individual such as this, mania may be manifested as frequent or continuous yelling or vocalizations which is very difficult to stop. It may also present as uncontrollable and ill-timed laughing, repetitive questions, or frequent interruptions in conversations. Manic speech is usually pressured, loud, very rapid, and difficult to interrupt. The speech can also contain disjointed thoughts.

3. *Elevated mood or irritability.* According to Sovner and Hurley (1986), in persons with an intellectual disability, hyperactivity is the thread connecting all of the associated symptoms of mania. They also note that the euphoric state of a person with an intellectual disability and mania is not as infectious as it can be in an individual without an intellectual disability (at least in the beginning of the manic phase). An elevation in mood for a person with an intellectual disability may be exhibited as laughing, giggling, smiling, or playfulness. The person may have difficulty respecting the personal boundaries of others. There may even be an increase in aberrant behaviors such as

self-injurious behavior which can be related to irritability the person may be experiencing. The person may also show signs of agitation such as pacing, aggression, restlessness, and a refusal to cooperate with requests.

4. *Decreased sleep.* One of the hallmark symptoms of bipolar disorder among individuals with and without an intellectual disability is a decreased need for sleep. They may awaken early, and there can be disruptive nighttime behaviors (e.g., pacing, vocalizations, agitation, inability to focus on an activity). This is particularly indicative if this is unusual for the person.

5. *Hedonistic activities.* One of the symptoms for Bipolar Disorder among the general population is excessive involvement in pleasurable activities with potentially high risk consequences. People with an intellectual disability may not have the opportunities or skills to engage in some of the typical behaviors exhibited by typically developed adults with this mood disorder (i.e., shopping sprees, driving fast, infidelities, drinking, etc.). Instead, they may exhibit this symptom by increased sexualized behavior, teasing peers, connecting with strangers on-line, binge eating, etc.

6. *Distractibility.* The individual may have difficulty attending to activities which were previously found pleasurable. For example, he or she is no longer able to watch a favorite television show for longer than a few seconds or minutes or the person may no longer be able to sustain attention to tasks on the job or at workshop.

One should be cautious about diagnosing Bipolar Disorder in an individual with an intellectual disability simply because the challenging behaviors tend to cycle. Cyclical behaviors are not necessarily evidence of a Bipolar Disorder. The behaviors may be suggestive of other mood disorders or anxiety. Cyclical behaviors can also occur in response to hormonal influences such as menstrual cycles, and in response to environmental changes or stressors. In diagnosing Bipolar Disorder, it is helpful to obtain information regarding family history of any mood disorders. It can also be very helpful to gather information on how the previous episodes of mania or hypomanic behavior presented themselves.

Mood disorder due to a general medical condition. It is important to rule out that a mood disorder is due to a general medical condition. Before any diagnosis is determined, a review of medical records should be undertaken, along with a medical evaluation. For example, the *DSM-IV-TR* lists the following disorders that mimic anxiety disorders: hyper- and hypothyroidism, cardiovascular conditions, respiratory conditions, and metabolic conditions. In order for a diagnosis of a Mood Disorder Due to a General Medical Condition to be given, it is "judged to be the direct physiological consequence of a general medical condition " (p. 181).

Anxiety Disorders

There is a wide variety of common anxiety disorders experienced by people with an intellectual disability. In addition, just as with the typically developing adult, when a person has one anxiety disorder, it is not uncommon to have another. Anxiety disorders tend to be underreported because the symptoms can be somewhat elusive. In the general population, the diagnosis of an anxiety disorder relies heavily on self-reports, the results of a structured mental status examination, and the observations of the clinician. For individuals who have an intellectual disability, feelings of anxiety may be exhibited through the emergence of unusual or challenging behaviors, not the self-report of anxiety or worry.

Generalized Anxiety Disorder. Generalized Anxiety Disorder (GAD) is characterized by excessive anxiety and worry about a number of events or activities (such as work or school performance), the individual finds it difficult to control the worry, and the anxiety and worry are associated with restlessness or feeling on edge, being easily fatigued, difficulty concentrating, irritability, muscle tension, and/or sleep disturbance (difficulty falling or staying asleep, or restless, unsatisfying sleep). The symptoms are similar for people with an intellectual disability. They may be restless, pace, or have difficulty sitting still. They may also repeat the same concern over and over because they are excessively worrying about something.

In a study by Favilla and Mucci (2000), they found that the experience of GAD in young adults with a mild intellectual disability largely paralleled the symptom presentation of individuals in the general population. They identified somatic complaints, rumination, and sleep disorders as the exceptions. An anxious individual with an intellectual disability will sometimes receive the label of being "very needy" or "attention-seeking." The individual may be requesting a lot of reassurance because he or she is worried about something or feeling a general sense of apprehension. Most people feel anxious at some time or another and the typical population tends to cope with feelings of anxiety by using cognitive strategies. These strategies are not usually effective for people with cognitive delays; therefore, they look to others to support them.

Anxiety and depression commonly co-occur. As with the general population, if anxiety is present, the presence of a depressive disorder should also be considered.

Panic Disorder. According to the *DSM-IV-TR*, the criteria for the diagnosis of a Panic Disorder includes unexpected panic attacks. In addition, at least one of the attacks has been followed by persistent concern about having further attacks or worry about the consequences of the attack (i.e., losing control, having a heart attack, etc.). Typical panic attacks can include a variety of symptoms such as, racing or pounding heart, sweating, trembling or shaking, shortness of breath, feeling of choking, chest pain or discomfort, nausea or abdominal distress, feeling dizzy, unsteady or faint, feeling unreal or detached, numbness or tingling sensation, chills or hot flashes, fear of dying, or fear of going crazy or losing control.

Panic attacks can occur during the day or night (i.e., nocturnal panic attacks). In fact, it is possible for panic attacks to occur only at night and not during the day. When they occur at night they are usually more difficult to diagnose because the person may attribute it to a nightmare or a night terror. With a non-verbal individual, there may be reports of sleep disturbances by the care providers. The individual may awaken during the night in a state of agitation and start to pace. He or she can also become aggressive and non-responsive to redirection. When considering a nocturnal panic attack, it is important to rule out any medical causes of such sleep disturbances. Some medical causes include possible sleep apnea, GI reflux, nocturnal angina, and nightmares. In addition, some psychotropic medications can produce abnormal dreams as a side effect – particularly with some of the antidepressant medication (Fuller & Sajatovic, 2002).

For a panic attack to be diagnosed, it must occur without an identified trigger. In other words, it must be unpredictable. Although some panic attacks can be situationally caused, to actually diagnose a panic disorder, some of the panic episodes must occur without any identifiable trigger.

Individuals with an **intellectual disability and Panic Disorder** may exhibit or experience atypical symptoms. An atypical presentation can occur because the person may lack the experience or ability to label the feelings, sensations, and emotions. Even with a person who is verbal, it may be difficult for the individual to explain what he or she experienced and was thinking. If the person is non-verbal then it can present as a behavioral issue. For example, social avoidance or agitation may suggest the possibility of an anxiety disorder.

Among individuals with an intellectual disability, a panic attack can be manifested in any of the following ways:

- Aggression
- Agitation; screaming; crying
- Reports of difficulty breathing and shallow breathing
- Physical complaints
- Resistance to going out in the community; wanting to stay at home and avoiding work
- Increased dependency needs
- History of 911 calls
- History of wanting to go to the hospital or frequent visits to nearby emergency rooms
- AWOL or running away from situations that worry them

Approximately 33% to 50% of individuals who have a panic disorder also have agoraphobia (*DSM-IV-TR*). *Agoraphobia* is a feeling of anxiety about being in places or situations from which escape might be difficult (or embarrassing). In addition, there is the feeling help may not be available in the event of having an unexpected or situationally predisposed panic attack. In the way this diagnosis is described in the *DSM-IV-TR*, the person must be able to predict the fear and plan to avoid it. This is not common for individuals with an intellectual disability. However, significant fear with leaving the home or going places may still be experienced. The reasons may just not be articulated. Agoraphobia in an individual with an intellectual disability may be suspected when the care providers or family members report the person no longer wants to go out into the community or to a day program. This can be misinterpreted as laziness. However, it may be a sign that the individual is starting to develop a pattern of avoidance and agoraphobic tendencies.

Obsessive-Compulsive Disorder. The essential features of Obsessive-Compulsive Disorder are recurrent obsessions or compulsions that are severe enough to be time-consuming or cause high levels of stress or impairment. Because these thoughts and behaviors can be common for a lot of people, a person is considered to have a disorder only when the obsessions or compulsions become severe, disabling, or time-consuming. Obsessive thoughts are unwanted thoughts that keep coming to mind and can provoke anxiety. Compulsions are urges that accompany the thoughts and can consist of the need to do or undo an activity. If the individual tries to resist the compulsion, it causes anxiety. The anxiety can be temporarily decreased if the individual acts upon the compulsion. The criteria for an Obsessive-Compulsive Disorder involve experiencing obsessive thoughts, compulsive behaviors, or both. Defining a recurrent thought as obsessive requires insight on the part of the person. Often individuals with an intellectual disability don't have that insight and have difficulty describing their thoughts in a way that would meet the criteria for "obsessive." It does not mean they don't have them, only that it is difficult to describe them. The *DSM-IV-TR* offers a specifier that notes "With Poor Insight," meaning the person does not recognize that the obsessions and compulsions are excessive or unreasonable. This can be a helpful distinction for individuals with an intellectual disability; however, it remains that they need to "communicate" their obsessive thoughts to identify them. It is more common that compulsive behavior is identified for the diagnosis to be applied. Compulsive behavior is observable by others, therefore, is more easily recognized.

What is a compulsive behavior?

- It is a repetitive behavior that the person feels driven to perform over and over again and cannot seem to stop.
- The behavior is largely irrational. It does not make sense.
- The behavior decreases anxiety and agitation. The person feels relief when the compulsion is completed.
- The behavior often increases with anxiety, frustration, or change.

Obsessive-Compulsive Disorder (OCD) can be overlooked and underdiagnosed among individuals with intellectual disability. Among this population, individuals may exhibit complex motor rituals, such as those associated with Tourette's disorder, which can be difficult to distinguish from OCD compulsions. The complex motor tics can look like obsessive-compulsive behaviors. For example, the individual can have tic-related symptoms which include rubbing, touching, tapping, stereotypical self-mutilation, staring, etc. It can be particularly difficult to differentiate between movement disorders, self-stimulatory behavior, and behaviors which are truly symptoms of OCD among individuals who are non-verbal. Some repetitive behaviors such as flicking light switches on and off, hoarding objects, and arranging furniture or other objects in the environment can all be indicators of OCD in individuals with an intellectual disability. OCD compulsions are usually preceded by anxiety and obsessional concerns. As discussed, obsessive concerns can be difficult to identify.

A better way to differentiate a tic from OCD compulsions is to learn how the person responds when the behavior is stopped. A person with a tic is more likely to show very little response, whereas, a person with an OCD compulsion is more likely to become agitated or anxious if he or she is not able to carry out the ritual.

In diagnosing this disorder among individuals with an intellectual disability, Gedye (1992) has constructed the Compulsive Behavior Checklist. This instrument lists 25 types of compulsions typical for individuals with an intellectual disability. This checklist does not conclusively result in a diagnosis of OCD but can be used as part of the assessment. According to Gedye (1992), the 25 compulsions are classified according to five categories which include ordering compulsions, completeness/incompleteness compulsions, cleaning compulsions, checking or touching, and deviant grooming compulsions.

With regard to ordering compulsions, the individual may insist on arranging items in a certain way or insist on placing objects in certain areas. If someone moves the item, the person may insist on returning it to the same place. This may even apply to rearranging where people are seated or standing. The individual may also be rigid in the adherence to routines or the order of activities.

With compulsions that involve completeness or incompleteness, an individual may repetitively complete and undo the task that was completed. For example, the person may dress and undress repeatedly, open and close doors, or empty shampoo bottles and other toileting containers in the bathroom.

If the individual is compulsive about cleanliness or tidiness, insistence on performing certain cleaning tasks excessively or performing them in a specific order may occur. This could also apply to daily hygiene activities in which the person washes certain body parts excessively.

An individual may also engage in grooming compulsions, including skin picking or picking at another part of the body to the extent it causes injury. The individual may also check in the mirror repetitively or pull on hair on the head or skin.

Posttraumatic Stress Disorder (PTSD). This is becoming one of the most prevalent disorders among individuals with dual diagnoses. It has been estimated that at least 60% of individuals with an intellectual disability have experienced some type of trauma, usually consisting of incidents of abuse (Sobsey, 1994). This statistic has been found to be higher depending on the study sample. It is proposed that the reason the statistics are so high for this population is because these individuals tend to be more dependent on care providers, which makes them more vulnerable. In addition, because some individuals with an intellectual disability cannot communicate well, they cannot expose the abuse to others.

Characteristic symptoms of PTSD as stated in the *DSM-IV-TR* are either the person experienced, witnessed, or was confronted with an event or events that involved actual or threatened death or serious injury, or the person experienced a threat to the physical integrity of self or others. Additionally, the person's response involved intense fear, helplessness, or horror. Moreover, the traumatic event is persistently re-experienced through intrusive thoughts and distressing recollections of the event. This includes distressing dreams, acting or feeling as if the event were reoccurring, intense psychological distress at exposure to internal or external cues that symbolize or resemble an aspect of the traumatic event, and/or physiological reactivity. The person experiences symptoms of increased arousal such as difficulty falling or staying asleep, irritability or outbursts of anger, difficulty concentrating, hypervigilance, and/or exaggerated startle response. In addition, avoidance of stimuli associated with the trauma is present. The individual may have an acute duration (symptoms of less than three months), chronic duration (symptoms present for three months or more), or delayed onset (onset of symptoms six months after the stressor). The above characteristics must be present to diagnose PTSD. It is important to note that everyone copes with trauma differently and not all people who experience a traumatic event develop a PTSD response to the event.

Diagnostic Considerations for Anxiety Disorders

The symptoms associated with anxiety disorders may also have other causes. Determining the accurate etiology can be difficult but is important. For example, anxiety may be caused by a variety of medical conditions. It can also be a symptom or byproduct of a substance use/abuse disorder. The expression of an anxiety disorder can also be influenced by the presence of a co-occurring mood disorder, environmental factors, psychosocial factors, or medications and their side effects. In addition, anxiety can be associated with a genetic syndrome. There are certain genetic syndromes that include behavioral patterns consistent with an anxiety disorder. Such syndromes include Prader-Willi syndrome which can be associated with OCD symptoms and Fragile X which can have accompanying anxiety (Szymanski & King, 1999). Therefore, it is also important to know whether a genetic disorder is contributing to the etiology of the symptoms.

Adjustment Disorder

The essential feature of an Adjustment Disorder is the development of clinically significant emotional or behavioral symptoms in response to an identifiable psychosocial stressor(s). The symptoms are present within three months of the onset of the stressor. Clinical significance of the reaction is indicated by either marked distress that is beyond what is expected or by impairment in social or occupational functioning. Subcategories of an Adjustment Disorder include Adjustment Disorder with depressed mood, anxiety, disturbance of conduct, and mixed disturbance of emotions and conduct.

Adjustment Disorders are quite common among individuals with mild and moderate intellectual disability since they may experience numerous environmental changes during their lives. They may also experience many losses, including changes in staff, family inconsistency, loss of residence due to discharge notices, loss of staff members, etc. Levitas and Hurley (2007) note in the *DM-ID* that "stressors for individuals with ID can include any need for an increase in autonomous functioning" (p. 501) such as a move to a new home or away from family, loss or change of an important caregiver, promotion to educational, vocational, or residential placement beyond one's comfort level, and onset of an illness. While these changes may not appear significant to others, they may be very stressful for the person experiencing them. The authors also note that marked distress may manifest as clinging, apparent loss of skills, withdrawal, irritability, aggression, self-injurious behavior, destructiveness, and loss of earlier compliance with care routines. If such symptoms develop, an Adjustment Disorder should be considered. While many of these changes can be viewed as positive by those working with the person, they can cause tremendous stress for the person. An Adjustment Disorder can develop whether the change is by the choice of the person (think of accepting a promotion, but feeling extremely anxious about the change) or by the choice of others (a staff person leaving, graduating from an educational program, needing to change residences, getting a new roommate, etc.).

Psychotic Disorders

Schizophrenia. According to the *DSM-IV-TR*, to meet the diagnostic criteria for schizophrenia, an individual needs to experience delusions, hallucinations, disorganized speech (e.g., frequent derailment or incoherence), very disorganized behavior or total lack of movement (catatonia), and/or negative symptoms (flat affect, inappropriate affect, poverty of speech or lack of initiated content, or lack of effort to act on one's behalf). The person needs to experience two or more of the symptoms for a significant portion of time during a one month period (or less if successfully treated).

According to the *DSM-IV-TR*, only one of these symptoms is required if "...delusions or hallucinations consist of a voice keeping up a running commentary on the person's behavior or thoughts, or two or more voices conversing with each other" (p. 312). Symptoms of schizophrenia are categorized as either "negative" or "positive." Negative symptoms include social isolation or withdrawal, loss of motivation, and a flat or inappropriate affect. Positive symptoms include delusions, hallucinations, and thought disorder. *Delusions* are strongly held, but incorrect beliefs that involve a misinterpretation of perceptions or experiences. *Hallucinations* can be experienced as auditory, olfactory, or visual. The individual may also taste or touch something that is not there. Auditory hallucinations are the most common form of hallucinations experienced by a person who is diagnosed as schizophrenic.

There are other psychotic disorders in which these signs and symptoms are present but to a different degree. It is very important to identify the appropriate disorder. The following chart may help with the distinction:

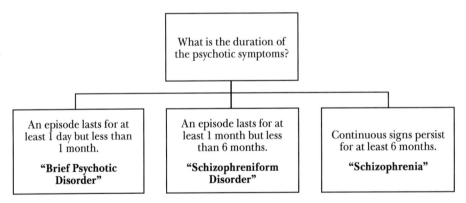

Differentiating between the different psychotic disorders may seem like a detail with little purpose; however, it is very important. Good or bad, when a diagnosis is given there are many assumptions made. For example, if a person is diagnosed with schizophrenia it is assumed it is a long-standing diagnosis. Therefore, it is less likely that medical conditions are ruled out, that other underlying causes for the symptoms are addressed, and that therapy is the recommended form of treatment. Instead, medication stabilization is assumed and medication is likely to focus on the psychosis as opposed to another emotional disorder. On the other hand, if it is identified as a Brief Psychotic Disorder, a thorough medical exam is typically conducted which includes ruling out a reaction to a substance (illegal and prescribed), a psychotic reaction to an emotional disorder, and a first psychotic episode. In addition, neurological syndromes are considered. More follow-up assessments are conducted to ensure appropriate care.

Because the symptoms and medical presentation of a person with an intellectual disability are often complicated, even a long-standing diagnosis of schizophrenia should be confirmed. Unfortunately, when a person cannot communicate clearly about his or her experience, past records become important. Often diagnoses remain in a person's records, and if a diagnosis is incorrect the treatment recommendations may be inappropriate and/or ineffective.

Delusional Disorder. A Delusional Disorder is characterized by non-bizarre delusions. The delusions may center around situations that occur in real life. The *DSM-IV-TR* provides examples of delusional beliefs such as being poisoned, loved at a distance, deceived by a spouse or lover, or having a disease. The behavior is not obviously bizarre or odd; however, it does have negative ramifications on the person's life.

It is imperative to consider the person's developmental level before diagnosing a Delusional Disorder. What may appear delusional for a typically developing adult may be developmentally appropriate for an adult with a developmental delay. Consider the following example:

A 40-year-old woman has a crush on a movie star. She wrote this person a letter and is very upset the person did not respond. She believes the person reads all of her letters and is shunning her on purpose.

This is highly unusual and age inappropriate for a typically developed adult. This response is delusional given her age and maturation. On the other hand, this is a typical presentation for a child in third to fifth grade. For a mildly to moderately delayed adult this response is not delusional, but appropriate given the person's developmental level.

Schizoaffective Disorder. Schizoaffective Disorder is characterized by an uninterrupted period of illness during which, at some time, there is either a Major Depressive Episode, a Manic Episode, or a Mixed Episode concurrent with symptoms of Schizophrenia. In addition, there have been delusions or hallucinations for at least two weeks in the absence of prominent mood symptoms. The primary characteristics are psychotic, the secondary characteristics are mood.

Among individuals with an intellectual disability who have been psychiatrically hospitalized, it is not uncommon to find a diagnosis of Schizoaffective Disorder. It appears to be an overused diagnosis and one that can be difficult to differentiate from other diagnoses. It is often mistakenly used for persons who suffer from a major depressive disorder with psychotic features, or a bipolar disorder with psychosis, particularly when the psychotic symptoms are not consistent with the mood presentation. Alternately, Schizoaffective Disorder can also be mistaken for schizophrenia since the individual may have experienced serious psychotic symptoms prior to the mood disturbance appearing. The mood disturbance may be overlooked and go untreated.

Schizoaffective Disorder can be identified by a process of lengthy observation of the individual and by an elimination of the other diagnostic categories. Since there is a need for longitudinal observation in making this diagnosis, it is not unusual for individuals to have had other diagnostic labels given prior to receiving this diagnosis. The following chart may help clarify the diagnostic distinctions.

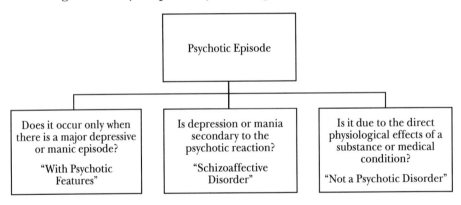

The diagnosis of a psychotic disorder among individuals with an intellectual disability can be difficult to make, particularly for individuals whose cognitive functioning lies within the severe to profound range. If an individual lacks the verbal skills to discuss delusional beliefs, one of the major criteria for the diagnosis of psychosis becomes difficult to detect. Even if the individual has expressive language skills, labeling and identifying subjective states may still be difficult. In addition, behavioral challenges sometimes seen in persons with a moderate or severe intellectual disability may be easily confused with behaviors associated with schizophrenia.

Examples include self-stimulatory behavior and a lack of socially appropriate interactions. Some behaviors characteristic of Autism may also appear similar to the symptoms sometimes seen in psychosis. Since approximately 70% of the people who have Autism also have a co-existing intellectual disability, it is important to consider this in the differential diagnosis. Individuals with Autism exhibit an unusual interpersonal style. In addition, they also may adopt various unusual gestures or postures in an attempt to alleviate some of the physical discomforts associated with sensory integration disorders. Caution should be applied so that sensory integration issues are not attributed to symptoms of psychosis.

Self-instructional talk exhibited sometimes by individuals with an intellectual disability should not be considered a sign of hallucinations. As part of the normal course of development, children may engage in fantasy play or talk to imaginary friends. Individuals with an intellectual disability may do the same. They may also engage in self-gratifying fantasies, which may resemble delusions when, in fact, they are nothing more than wishful thinking. Therefore, any delusions in persons with an intellectual disability should first be considered as possible fantasy.

The following are some possible indicators that an individual with an intellectual disability may be suffering from a psychotic disorder:

Delayed responses. Individuals who are responding to internal stimuli (i.e., voices in their heads) may appear to be very distracted and take longer to respond to conversations.

When they do respond, their responses may not be appropriate or the content of their responses may be very tangential and not coherent.

Agitation. If the individual is experiencing auditory of visual hallucinations, the person may appear agitated, anxious, or confused. The agitation could lead to an increase in aggressive behaviors or self-injurious behaviors.

Inappropriate affect. The individual may be found laughing or displaying an emotion that is not congruent with the conversation or the activity.

Sleep disturbances. The individual may find it difficult to go to sleep because of hearing voices or feeling agitated.

Talking to themselves. If the individual is talking to him or herself and having a conversation with no apparent person it could be a response to auditory hallucinations. However, this should be distinguished from self-talk that is instructional or self-soothing.

Staring. The person may stare off into space or nod as though involved in a conversation or listening to a conversation that is not audible to others.

Covering eyes or ears. The individual may cover his or her eyes or ears as if trying to shut out certain stimuli. Caution should be applied when interpreting this behavior as this can also be an indication of anxiety or a response to physical pain.

Shadow boxing/Odd posturing. If the individual shows odd posturing it can be reflective of psychosis. However, caution should be applied as it may also be reflective of other conditions. For example, odd posturing can occur as a medication-related side effect or in response to an Obsessive-Compulsive Disorder. It may also be a movement disorder that is neurologically driven or reflective of a Stereotypic Movement Disorder which consists of non-functional repeated movements.

Suspiciousness around food. The person may even stop eating. This can signal paranoia, a delusion that the food is contaminated or poisoned. It can also suggest olfactory/gustatory hallucinations.

A decline in self-help skills. The individual's self-care skills may decline. The person may no longer want to perform them or may be considerably less thorough in completely them.

Fearfulness and social withdrawal. The person may have this reaction to friends or family. The person may also become more socially withdrawn than is typical for the person.

Wearing multiple layers of clothing. This can be a result of the sense of disintegration experienced by individuals with psychosis. This should be interpreted with caution for individuals who have lived on the streets or in institutions where protecting belongings is an important part of life. It can also be a symptom of sensorimotor integration deficits or a symptom of a medical condition, such as hypothyroidism, which results in the individual feeling cold.

Ryan (1996) has suggested some guidelines to help identify whether a person who is non-verbal and exhibiting unusual behaviors may be experiencing hallucinations or delusions. First, determine the rationality of the behavior. Does the individual's behavior make sense in the context of his or her life? For example, the individual may have imaginary friends because he lacks a social support network and he is lonely. Consequently, he engages in some imaginary interactions to appease his loneliness and boredom. Second, obtain information regarding the existence of psychiatric disorders in the family. Is there a history of schizophrenia or psychosis among any relatives or immediate family members? Third, assess the course of the symptoms. Is the behavior unusual? Does it come and go over time?

Ryan (2001) has also identified symptoms that are almost never indications of psychosis. These include the following:

1. Volitional self-talk
2. Vocal tics such as those that occur with Tourette's disorder
3. Behavior that is the result of modeling or imitating other individuals
4. Phenomena that the individual can control and start and stop at will

In making diagnostic distinctions of the individual's symptoms, it is extremely important to rule out any underlying medical causes for the psychosis. This becomes particularly important for individuals who do not possess the verbal skills to communicate their experience. For example, metabolic disorders, endocrine disorders, substance use, neurological damage, nutritional deficiencies, and infections are some medical diagnostic possibilities when the individual is presenting with psychotic symptoms (First and Tasman, 2004). In addition, some sensory deficits can be mistaken for unusual behaviors seen in psychosis. For example, an individual who bats out with his or her hands may be thought to be responding to visual hallucinations when, in fact, he or she has uncorrected myopia. The individual who waves her fingers in front of her eyes may be experiencing a headache rather than a hallucination. Gustatory and olfactory hallucinations can also occur with complex partial seizures (Neppe & Tucker, 1988).

Personality Disorders

Personality can be defined as a dynamic and organized set of characteristics possessed by a person that uniquely influences his or her cognitions, motivations, and behaviors in various situations (http://www.wikipedia.com/Personalitypsychology). It arises from within the individual and remains fairly consistent throughout life. According to the *DSM-IV-TR*, personality disorders are defined by an enduring pattern of inner experience and behavior that deviates markedly from expectations of the individual's culture. This pattern is manifested in *cognition* (i.e., ways of perceiving and interpreting self, other people, and events), *affectivity* (i.e., range, intensity, lability, and appropriateness of emotional response), *interpersonal functioning,* and *impulse control.*

Diagnosing individuals with an intellectual disability as having a personality disorder has been somewhat controversial. First, any time you see the word "cognition" or "motivation" you know that it will be very important to consider the developmental level of the person. It cannot be assumed that the cognitive processes such as decision making, judgment, and perceptions are going to be the same for a person with an intellectual disability as for a typically developed adult. In addition, the motivation and intention of behaviors are often much different. Second, what may be considered inappropriate or deviating "markedly from expectations of the individual's culture" for a typically developed adult, may not be inappropriate for the developmental level of a person with an intellectual disability. The authors of the Personality Disorders chapter in the *DM-ID* state "Individuals with ID are likely to experience a delayed development that may result in an immature or a less completely developed personality, which will have traits or features of a personality disorder" (Lindsay, Dana, Dosen, Gabriel & Young, 2007, p. 313).

A diagnosis of a personality disorder is essentially a historical diagnosis. There needs to be evidence of a long standing rigid pattern of thoughts and behaviors that can be traced to at least adolescence or early adulthood. In addition, the behavior patterns need to be stable over time, pervasive, and inflexible.

The *DSM-IV-TR* lists ten personality disorders which are divided into clusters. There are eleven categories in all, with one category listed as Personality Disorder, Not Otherwise Specified. The *DSM-IV-TR* classifies the disorders as falling in one of three clusters. The clustering system has been criticized because the characterizations are often generalizations. Also, individuals frequently present with co-occurring personality disorders that fall in different clusters. This causes professionals to question the practical use of the clusters. For each of the personality disorders the person needs to meet the criteria for three, four, or five of the characteristics listed. This section will include a brief description of the disorders. However, please refer to the *DSM-IV-TR* for the specific criteria. The three clusters are:

Cluster A (odd or eccentric disorders)
- Paranoid Personality Disorder
- Schizoid Personality Disorder
- Schizotypal Personality Disorder

Cluster B (dramatic, emotional, or erratic disorders)
- Antisocial Personality Disorder
- Borderline Personality Disorder

- Histrionic Personality Disorder
- Narcissistic Personality Disorder

Cluster C (anxious or fearful disorders)
- Avoidant Personality Disorder
- Dependent Personality Disorder
- Obsessive-Compulsive Personality Disorder (not the same as Obsessive-Compulsive Disorder)

Symptoms characteristic of the personality disorders in the general, adult population also apply to individuals with an intellectual disability. It is up to the professionals working with the individual to assess the degree his or her cognitive ability determines how closely the symptoms resemble the ones applied to the general population as defined by *DSM-IV-TR*. In general, clinicians are challenged in diagnosing these conditions among individuals with a severe or profound intellectual disability. Some clinicians have suggested that personality disorder diagnoses should not be given to individuals functioning below the mild level of intellectual disability (Dana, 1993).

Cluster A Personality Disorders
Individuals with a Cluster A Personality Disorder may appear odd or eccentric. The *Paranoid Personality Disorder* is when the person is very suspicious and mistrusting. These individuals assume others are going to cause them harm or deceive them. Individuals with a *Schizoid Personality Disorder* present with a restricted range of emotions or flat affect and detach from social relationships. Individuals with *Schizotypal Personality Disorder* tend to have unusual behavior patterns that include social deficits, odd beliefs, excessive social anxiety, and suspicious ideation.

When considering a Cluster A Personality Disorder for a person with an intellectual disability, other diagnoses such as Pervasive Developmental Disorder, psychotic disorders, and anxiety disorders must be ruled out. One of the complicating factors of identifying a person with intellectual as having a Cluster A Personality Disorder is that with this population, the behavioral characteristics that can appear odd, suspicious, or avoidant may very well be a pattern of the intellectual disability and not a personality disorder.

Cluster B Personality Disorders

The personality disorders that generally get the most attention are those falling in Cluster B (Antisocial, Borderline, Histrionic, and Narcissistic Personality Disorder). People with Cluster B disorders often appear dramatic, emotional, or erratic. Individuals with these disorders tend to have the most challenges with relationships; therefore, living situations are often unstable. The person is more emotionally labile and tends to react the most with unsafe behavior (threaten to harm self or others). Because individuals with these personality disorders can be a safety risk, they receive a lot of time, energy, and focus from the professionals working with them.

Borderline Personality Disorder (BPD). This disorder is marked by a pattern of instability in interpersonal relationships, self-image, and emotions, as well as marked impulsivity. You may see a person who cries easily and often, threatens self-harm, attempts to engage in self-harm or self-mutilation, is easily angered, threatens to leave the facility or move out, has irrational ideas about relationships with others, and perseverates on the same issues. Individuals with a borderline organization to their personality have a lack of anxiety tolerance. Under stress they can regress and act impulsively. They can be high functioning in some areas and extremely low functioning in other areas. Individuals with this personality disorder typically see the world in black or white terms. This is their attempt to provide order and structure to their internal world.

The characteristics of BPD in the general population and those for individuals with an intellectual disability are similar. One of the salient features of this disorder is a frantic effort to avoid real or imagined abandonment. It is also common for individuals with BPD to engage in inappropriate social behavior with others as a means of interacting or connecting, such as crossing personal or physical boundaries. They may resort to desperate and unsafe measures to keep people close.

Histrionic Personality Disorder. This disorder is marked by a pattern of excessive emotionality and attention-seeking. It is characterized by discomfort in situations where the person is not the center of attention. The person may attempt to gain attention by inappropriate and/or sexually seductive behavior, dramatic and exaggerated emotional expression, and use of physical appearance to draw attention to self. The person may also exhibit a style of speech that lacks detail, rapidly shifting and shallow expression of emotions, tendency to be easily influenced by others, and/or the impression that there is greater intimacy than there really is in relationships.

The *DSM-IV-TR* notes there is a higher rate of Somatization and Conversion Disorders as well as other personality disorders for individuals with Histrionic Personality Disorder. The characteristics of this disorder are often played out in relationships. The *DSM-IV-TR* also suggests that individuals with this profile may act out a role, such as "the princess," "the victim," "the martyr," etc. This dramatic characterization is typically the most prominent characteristic and one that is easily identifiable.

Antisocial Personality Disorder. Individuals with Antisocial Personality Disorder are characterized by a pervasive pattern of "disregard for and violation of the rights of others" (*DSM-IV-TR*, p. 701). This can be seen in a failure to conform to the law, deceitfulness, impulsivity, irritability or aggressiveness, disregard for the safety of others, irresponsibility, and/or lack of remorse. This is a very difficult disorder to diagnose for individuals with intellectual disability. The main reason is because many of the other psychiatric disorders present as "impulsive," "irritable," "aggressive," and "irresponsible" for this population. In addition, these individuals often don't have the opportunity to break the law and may not understand the consequences if they do. For these reasons this diagnosis is infrequently given to individuals with an intellectual disability. If the diagnosis is given, it should be carefully assessed for its appropriateness.

Narcissistic Personality Disorder. Individuals with Narcissistic Personality Disorder are characterized by a pattern of grandiosity, need for admiration, and lack of empathy. Individuals with this disorder exhibit a sense of entitlement, appear arrogant or haughty, believe they are "special" and unique, and are often envious of others or believe others are envious of them. This is another disorder that is not often suggested for individuals with an intellectual disability. Individuals with an intellectual disability are often more needy of attention than typically developing adults. This is not the same as a person with a Narcissistic Personality Disorder. In addition, it is difficult to identify to what extent fantasies are developmentally appropriate or narcissistic in nature. In general, caution needs to be used when considering this diagnosis for a person with an intellectual disability.

Cluster C Personality Disorders

When considering whether a person meets the criteria for a Cluster C personality disorder, the main challenge is ruling out other disorders that may present similarly. In general the Cluster C disorders are characterized by a person who is anxious or fearful. A person with an *Avoidant Personality Disorder* tends to avoid activities that involve a lot of interpersonal interaction and appears reserved or inhibited in social situations, shows restraint in relationships, and is reluctant to take risks and try new things. The characteristics of this disorder include an avoidance of social interactions which can be misinterpreted as autistic-like traits. These two disorders are differentiated by the reason the person is avoidant of these situations. The individual with an Avoidant Personality Disorder is very fearful of rejection. Consequently, he or she avoids interpersonal situations for fear of criticism and negative results, even though he or she has a desire for that social contact. A person with autism is more likely to avoid interpersonal situations as a personal preference, as opposed to fear.

A person with a *Dependent Personality Disorder* tends to have difficulty making everyday decisions, looks to others for advice or guidance before doing anything, appears insecure, feels uncomfortable being alone, and is unlikely to disagree with someone. The descriptions of this disorder may be more likely for persons with an intellectual disability, not because of a pervasive personality trait, but because of their circumstances, past experiences, and messages they are receiving from their caregivers. If they are living in a supervised home setting and are not offered the opportunities for independence, they may feel very unsure about the challenges of being more independent. Their living situation may be set up in a way that they are required to ask for permission before doing something. This promotes the tendency to ask for advice and guidance before doing something. In addition, if they are dually diagnosed with co-existing mental health disorders, this response may be very reasonable because of the confusion about their experiences and how to cope with them.

The third Cluster C personality disorder is *Obsessive-Compulsive Personality Disorder (OCPD)*. Individuals with OCPD tend to be extremely focused on order and routine, may appear perfectionistic, rigid, and stubborn, and/or may be inflexible about some matters. At the same time, this is differentiated from an Obsessive-Compulsive Disorder (OCD) in that OCPD overlaps more with a "Type A" personality (*DSM-IV-TR*), and OCD is more indicative of an irrational routine or ritual that is associated with a compulsive thought. Individuals with OCPD tend to exhibit the characteristics as a lifestyle, as opposed to knowing it is irrational and wanting to stop. Another characteristic of some people with OCPD is hoarding. If you are working with an individual who has lived in group homes, institutions, or on the streets, hoarding may be a lifestyle of survival and should not be considered deviant from the norm.

The *DSM-IV-TR* also contains a category for behavioral patterns that do not match these ten disorders but nevertheless have the characteristics of a personality disorder. This category is labeled Personality Disorder, Not Otherwise Specified. It is also possible for individuals to receive a diagnosis of more than one personality disorder.

Gathering an extensive background and history on any individual when considering a personality disorder is extremely important but it is even more so if the person has an intellectual disability. Often the person's experience is such that the response is reasonable and expected, even when it appears socially inappropriate. Because personality disorders often significantly impact relationships, the history of attachments and living situations is essential to consider. If the person has lived in various places, had only short-term relationships, has no family involvement, and has not felt safe, the need for attention and feelings of insecurity, fear, and irritability are reasonable. Rather than simply looking to see if the behavior patterns meet the criteria, consider the behavior patterns developmentally and within the context of the person's history and experiences.

Impulse Control Disorders

Most of the Impulse Control Disorders are easy to classify because they are characterized by distinct behavior patterns, such as *Kleptomania, Pyromania, Pathological Gambling,* and *Trichotillomania.* Part of the diagnosis is that individuals engage in these behaviors despite the negative impact it is having on their life. There is some controversy about the degree that persons with an intellectual disability engages in the behavior despite their awareness of the negative consequences. However, these disorders are not often confused with other disorders and they descriptively designate a behavioral challenge.

Intermittent Explosive Disorder. The more commonly diagnosed Impulse Control Disorder is Intermittent Explosive Disorder (IED). According to the *DSM-IV-TR*, IED is characterized by experiencing several discrete episodes of failure to resist aggressive impulses that result in serious assaultive acts or destruction of property. The degree of aggressiveness expressed during the episodes is grossly out of proportion to any precipitating psychosocial stressors. The aggressive episodes are not better accounted for by another mental health disorder and are not due to the direct physiological effects of a substance (e.g., a non-prescription drug, a medication) or a general medical condition.

This diagnosis tends to be given to individuals with an intellectual disability who exhibit aggressive behaviors when the etiology of the aggression remains unclear. In the general population the prevalence rate of this diagnosis is very low, and there is no data to show this is more common for individuals with an intellectual disability. It should not be assumed that aggressive incidents are reflective of IED. The *DM-ID* notes Intermittent Explosive Disorder "may have greater validity for individuals with Mild ID because clinicians can better judge the discontinuity between stress and aggressive behavior" (Rifkin & Barnhill, 2007, p. 292).

A diagnosis of IED is really a diagnosis of exclusion. Aggression can occur as a result of several different psychiatric conditions. Impulsive aggression can occur during the course of a mood disorder, especially during a manic phase of Bipolar Disorder. It can also occur during the course of an agitated depressive episode or it may appear as a variant of Obsessive-Compulsive Disorder (OCD). This disorder should also be differentiated from a personality change due to a general medical condition, substance intoxication or withdrawal, delirium or dementia. It can also be an associated feature of Schizophrenia in which it may occur in response to hallucinations or delusions. It can also be the result of a rage attack that can be seen in individuals who have Tourette's disorder. These diagnoses should be considered and excluded before a diagnosis of IED is given.

When assessing for the presence of an Impulse Control Disorder the following medical tests can rule out other causes:

- Blood and urine toxicology screens may reveal the use of other substances.
- Partial complex seizures and focal brain lesions may be evaluated by use of an EEG.
- Brain imaging may further clarify contributing neurological structure.
- Hypoglycemia, a rare cause of impulsive aggression, may be detected by blood chemistry screen.

Attention Deficit/Hyperactivity Disorder

The essential feature of Attention-Deficit/Hyperactivity Disorder is a persistent pattern of inattention and/or hyperactivity that is more frequent and severe than is expected for an individual at a comparable level of development. The symptoms may manifest in academic, occupational, or social situations. The characteristics of hyperactivity and impulsivity are more likely to be identified for a person with an intellectual disability. For example, the characteristics of inattention are more difficult to observe because they are already common in individuals with an intellectual disability.

The DSM-IV-TR describes inattention as:
1. Fails to give close attention to details
2. Often has difficulty sustaining attention in tasks and play activities
3. Often does not seem to listen when spoken to
4. Often does not follow through on instructions and fails to finish schoolwork, chores, or duties in the workplace
5. Often has difficulty organizing tasks and activities
6. Often avoids, dislikes, or is reluctant to engage in tasks that require sustained mental effort
7. Often loses things necessary for tasks or activities
8. Is often easily distracted by outside stimuli
9. Is often forgetful in daily activities

The DSM-IV-TR describes hyperactivity as:
1. Often fidgets with hands or feet or squirms in a seat or chair
2. Often leaves seat in situations in which remaining seated is expected
3. Often runs about or climbs excessively, or, in adults, a feeling of restlessness occurs
4. Often has difficulty playing or engaging in activities quietly
5. Is often "on the go" or acts like they are "driven by a motor"
6. Often talks excessively

The *DSM-IV-TR* describes impulsivity as:
1. Often blurts out answers before questions are completed
2. Often has difficulty awaiting turn
3. Often interrupts or intrudes on others conversations or activities

The primary characteristics that define this disorder are related to executive functioning. As noted in this book, executive functioning is an area of neurological functioning that is frequently impacted for individuals with an intellectual disability. Therefore, it can be challenging to identify ADHD because of the overlap of symptoms with an intellectual disability that includes a short attention span, impulsivity, etc. There are also several medical conditions that can mimic the symptoms, such as various neurological disorders or endocrine disorders.

According to a study by Feinstein and Reiss (1996), the actual prevalence of ADHD in this population is similar to the rate among the general population which is estimated to be between 4% and 11%. The criteria must be evaluated in light of the individual's developmental level and in light of any syndromes the individual may have. While diagnosing ADHD for a person with an intellectual disability can be difficult, it is a very important component of a treatment plan. If a person is dually diagnosed with intellectual disability and ADHD, accommodations will need to address organization, planning, decision making, and independent living. For example, someone with a mild level of intellectual disability has the cognitive skills to self-administer and manage medication. On the other hand, if ADHD is also present, remembering to take the medication and keeping the prescription filled is going to be much more of a challenge. If ADHD is not addressed, it can be very frustrating for the individual as well as those working with him or her.

Sleep Disorders

Sleep disorders have been frequently overlooked in working with individuals with an intellectual disability. However, disruptions of sleep are common among this population. As noted by Espie (2000), "Mental retardation represents a small and neglected corner of sleep medicine. However, disruption of sleep architecture and sleep-wake rhythms appears to be common in this population, particularly in those with severe underlying brain damage" (p. 507). He further notes that unregulated sleep-wake cycles can have a relationship to behavioral challenges among individuals with an intellectual disability.

Sleep is a relatively complex process that involves phases and stages which vary depending on the age of the person and other individual factors. However, it conforms to patterns. Some people may need nine hours of sleep per night, while others may only need six. In addition, some people may fall into a deep sleep more quickly than others. Despite these differences, the stages are relatively consistent. Stage 1 and stage 2 are comprised of a light sleep, whereas stage 3 and 4 represent more of a deep sleep. Rapid eye movement sleep (REM) occurs in cycles throughout the night. Typically, the first episode of REM occurs around 70-90 minutes after the individual has fallen asleep. There is some variance about this time frame. In addition, there is some emerging research to suggest that sleep staging in individuals with severe brain damage may not conform to the conventional staging patterns. For example, Richdale, Cotton, and Hibbit (1999) report a greater likelihood of past and current sleep difficulties with individuals with Prader-Willi syndrome (PWS). They also found a greater likelihood of excessive daytime sleepiness among their sample of individuals with PWS.

For individuals with or without an intellectual disability, the importance of a good night's sleep cannot be emphasized enough. Sleep deprivation can lead to an increase in psychiatric symptoms, and it can compromise immune functioning. According to Stiefel (2007), sleep disorders among individuals with an intellectual disability should be considered if any of the following conditions are present:

- The individual is presenting with severe behavioral problems
- Severe snoring is noted
- There is excessive daytime fatigue
- The individual is taking psychotropic medications, particularly several medications of the same class
- Late afternoon fatigue is observed
- Changes are noted in the individual's functioning level
- Morning is a difficult time for the individual

The following decision tree is provided to aid in the differential diagnosis of chronic insomnia versus other sleep disorders.

Step 1: Evaluate the medical condition as a possible underlying cause of the insomnia.

Does the individual's history and medical status suggest an underlying medical disorder? Genetic syndromes should not be overlooked since sleep disorders can occur among a variety of syndromes, including Tourette's disorder, Fragile X, Prader-Willi, Angelman's syndrome, Turners syndrome, and Marfan syndrome, etc.

Medical conditions that can impact sleep include pain related conditions such as arthritis, gastroesophageal reflux, congestive heart failure, sleep apnea, chronic obstructive pulmonary disease, osteoporosis, and Parkinson's disease.

Step 2: Evaluate for the possibility of an underlying psychiatric disorder.

Is there evidence that the individual is experiencing a significant amount of anxiety or symptoms of a mood disorder? Sleep disturbances can occur with depression, anxiety disorders, ADHD, psychotic disorders, and among the bipolar spectrum. They may also occur with PTSD, since a hallmark symptom can be nightmares. The individual may be afraid to fall asleep for fear of experiencing the nightmares again.

Step 3: Evaluate for possible drug related insomnia.

Is the individual taking sedatives, hypnotics, alcohol, or other drugs? The use of drugs and alcohol can have a significant impact on a person's sleep stages. In addition, side effects of prescribed medications can include disruptions in sleep patterns.

Step 4: Evaluate for possible circadian rhythm disorder and for poor sleep hygiene.

Is the sleep normal but occurring at the wrong time? Sometimes an individual may be sleeping several hours at a time and completing the typical sleep cycles, although they are sleeping during the day. This can be a side effect of the medication. This may also occur because the person is staying up late at night and is fatigued during the day. For example, a person is living in a group home and knows staff will provide a lot of attention during the overnight hours when everyone else is asleep. The person will be less motivated to be awake during the day and will be fatigued because of the nighttime activity. This can result in a disrupted sleep schedule.

Step 5: Evaluate for possible sleep apnea.

Does the individual snore or exhibit irregular breathing patterns when sleeping? Sleep apnea is a very common cause of sleep disturbance. This needs to be evaluated at a sleep clinic because most often the person is not aware of this difficulty. The person may report being fatigued even after a full night of sleep. However, the apnea disrupts the ability to benefit from the deeper stages of sleep. The person is unable to feel rested.

Dementia

Currently, the frequency of dementia in individuals with an intellectual disability remains unknown. The course of any dementia depends upon its cause. There are some dementias which are potentially reversible, including those caused by medications, depression, or metabolic disorders. However, most dementias have historically been considered progressive with some evidence to suggest that early treatment may slow down the process, particularly with dementia of the Alzheimer's type. Consequently, it is important to be aware of the possibility of dementia among older individuals with an intellectual disability so that appropriate supports can be provided. In considering whether or not a dementia process is present the following questions should be asked:

1. Has there been a change over time in the individual's skill level including self-care skills?
2. Has there been a decline in participation in activities the person used to find pleasurable?
3. Is there a depression present which may present as a pseudodementia?
4. Is there a family history of dementia?
5. What is the individual's medical history including current health status?
6. Has the individual manifested any gait disturbances or movement disorders?
7. Has a mental status evaluation been conducted, but modified in response to the individual's level of cognitive functioning?
8. Have any specialized tests been done including an MRI or CT scan, or any specialized laboratory tests, along with routine laboratory tests?

Chapter 4

Medical Contributors to Psychiatric Conditions

Before reaching a conclusion that a behavior is the result of a psychiatric issue, it is important to ensure it is not the result of an underlying medical condition. This is important because there are various medical conditions that can present as psychiatric symptoms. Consequently, this chapter addresses the need to have a comprehensive medical examination as part of an assessment process. This becomes particularly important when working with individuals with intellectual disorders who do not possess the verbal skills to communicate symptoms such as a racing heart or tingling sensations.

When establishing a symptom profile for a person with an intellectual disability, traditional interviews might be insufficient. Adapted tools to help with communication can be very helpful. For example, one way is to use pictures that show a happy or hurt facial expression while pointing to different parts of the person's body. The person can point to the facial expression as the doctor or nurse points to each part of the body. The doctor begins with the fingers, hand, wrist, arm, etc. Sometimes when talking to an authority figure, a person may agree with everything the doctor suggests because the person thinks that is expected. Therefore, include such questions as, "How does your hair (toe, fingernail, etc.) feel?" as a discriminating comparison.

With someone who has an intellectual disability, the first sign of illness may be a change in behavior. Often, the person's behavioral challenges may be attributed to willfulness, attention-seeking, or manipulative intentions. Therefore, underlying medical conditions can be overlooked. The following are some indicators that a behavior may be related to an underlying medical issue:

- The person exhibits pain-related behaviors either through changes in facial expressions, body positions, or movements. For example, a person may show facial grimacing when changing positions or may limp after walking longer distances.
- Changes in weight, particularly significant losses in weight, may indicate an underlying medical issue. Therefore, it is very important to monitor weight trends.
- The individual may exhibit the same behaviors that were exhibited with a previous illness. If an individual has a history of a particular medical condition, it is helpful to know the signs the person demonstrated when first diagnosed with the illness.
- There may be changes in sleep due to pain or discomfort.
- If the individual has a medical condition that is progressive, it can be anticipated that the person will eventually experience physical discomfort or increasing discomfort.
- The person may engage in self-injurious behavior that is directed to a specific part of the body.
- There may be a change in the individual's vital signs.
- There may be a recent or sudden change in the person's behavior.
- The individual has an aversion to wearing certain clothes or shoes.
- Changes in ambulation may occur. For example, the person develops an unsteady gait or has had recent falls.
- The person may show a sensitivity to being touched on certain parts of the body.
- The individual maintains odd postures while lying down or while sitting.
- The person exhibits the behavior across environments and with a variety of people.
- The behavior occurs in cycles such as pain related to menses.
- There is a sudden increase or decrease in energy level. The individual may want to spend more time in bed or be constantly moving.
- There is a change in the individual's mental status or mental alertness. The individual may seem more confused.

- There are obvious signs of a change in one or more of the individual's medical systems, such as a change in elimination, changes in breathing, etc.
- The behavioral challenges do not appear to be linked to any trigger in the environment. For example, the person starts banging his head for no apparent reason.
- The individual may cry, moan, or groan.
- The person complains of being in pain or discomfort.
- The individual has identified medical conditions that require frequent monitoring.

Obtaining a family history of medical conditions can be helpful. Since there can be a genetic predisposition to some medical conditions, it is helpful to know what conditions have been present in other family members. This can assist in identifying underlying medical causes of behaviors and psychiatric symptoms.

Medical Contributors and Behavioral Challenges

When confronted with behavioral challenges, note the area of the body that is involved. This may provide clues as to whether or not a medical issue is involved. If someone is engaging in self-injurious behavior, is it localized to one area? For example, if the person is hitting her ear, then it would be logical to rule out a physical issue in that location, such as an ear infection. To help identify more details about the symptoms, the following considerations may be helpful:

- Is there a specific area of the body involved which could indicate a disease process in that particular location? Does the individual always target that area?
- Consider how pain from some of the more common medical conditions are experienced and displayed by others. For example, if someone has arthritis it may be manifested by a resistance to getting up. The individual may resist walking around or may be slow to move. The person may also just want to sit down as the pain increases or drop to the floor as an indication of discomfort.
- Consider if you were non-verbal, what would you be trying to communicate if you were in physical discomfort or favoring a certain area of your body?

Common Medical Conditions in Individuals with an Intellectual Disability

Since it is very important to assess for possible medical contributors to any psychiatric condition, the following is a list of medical conditions that have been frequently encountered among this population.

1. **Gastrointestinal conditions.** Gastrointestinal difficulties are common in individuals with developmental conditions (DeVeer, Bos, Boer, Bohmer, & Francke, 2008).

Dysphagia. When working with individuals with an intellectual disability, it is helpful for care providers to have a basic knowledge of some of the risk factors and signs that the individual may be experiencing swallowing difficulties. If these difficulties remain undetected, there is a greater risk of morbidity and mortality due to incidents of aspiration pneumonia and deaths due to choking.

Physical risk factors for dysphagia (i.e., swallowing difficulties) can include cerebral palsy, malformations of the face, missing teeth, neuromuscular disorders such as Parkinson's syndrome, poor motor skills, Down syndrome, gastrointestinal reflux, and seizures disorders. Dysphagia can result from conditions that produce decreased motor coordination or conditions that cause some type of structural obstruction with regard to swallowing.

The following are some warning signs that an individual may have swallowing difficulties:

- There is a pattern of continued weight loss.
- The individual may have reoccurring pneumonia and respiratory infections. The pneumonia may have been aspiration pneumonia versus viral or bacterial pneumonia.
- There may be behavioral issues around mealtimes, including taking longer to eat, resistiveness around eating, throwing food, spilling food, turning away from the food, and a general refusal to eat.
- The individual experiences obvious difficulties chewing.
- Coughing can be observed during mealtimes.
- Episodes of choking or gagging can occur during meals.
- Sometimes there are no overt signs with an individual who is a silent aspirator until a fever is present or the person becomes lethargic.

To identify dysphagia, evaluations or more detailed medical procedures, such as a swallow study, may be needed. Changes in the individual's ability to swallow may necessitate dietary modifications. Depending upon the degree of dysphagia, the texture of the diet may need to be changed to include such modifications as a pureed or a ground diet. The consistency of the liquids may also need to be modified. Caretakers may need to alter feeding techniques, such as ensuring the meal is presented in bite sized pieces. Modifications may also include repositioning the individual, decreasing environmental distractions during meals, or providing enhanced supervision during mealtimes.

In addition to certain physical conditions increasing the likelihood of swallowing difficulties among this population, iatrogenic factors such as medication-related side effects may impact the ability to swallow. Some psychotropic medications, including the novel anti-psychotics, have a potential side effect of producing dysphagia by destroying the cilia that line the esophagus (Fuller & Sajatovic, 2002). Any sedating medications (e.g., anticonvulsants, sedatives) have the potential to contribute to dysphagia (Fuller & Sajatovic, 2002).

Behavioral issues can also increase the risk of choking. These behaviors include eating too rapidly and overstuffing food in the mouth. Stealing food from others and eating it too quickly can also pose a choking hazard. Food stealing can be particularly problematic if the individual is on a special textured diet such as a ground diet. While food stealing appears to be more commonly seen in individuals who have been institutionalized, it can also occur in people who have increased appetites from medications (Fuller & Sajatovic, 2002).

The importance of observing behaviors at mealtimes cannot be overstated. An increased level of monitoring and awareness around eating for all individuals with an intellectual disability will help to ensure their continued safety and well-being. Although difficulties with swallowing can range from mild to severe cases of dysphagia, these difficulties can spiral into deteriorating health conditions if not properly identified, treated, and managed.

Gastroesophageal reflux (GERD). Gastrointestinal problems which include diarrhea, gastritis, gastroesophageal reflux, chronic inflammation of the digestive tract, lactase deficiencies, and constipation can all cause discomfort that can trigger behavioral problems. Any of these issues can impact an individual's behavior because they can produce pain.

Gastoesophageal reflux disease (GERD) is a common condition of the gastrointestinal tract which often occurs among individuals with an intellectual disability (DeVeer et al., 2008). Predisposing factors for gastroesophageal reflux include cerebral palsy, non-ambulatory status, scoliosis, the use of anticonvulsive medications, and the severity of the intellectual disability (DeVeer et al., 2008). DeVeer et al. (2008) found that individuals whose cognitive functioning abilities were within the moderate to severe ranges of an intellectual disability had more incidents of GERD than those functioning within the higher ranges.

Reflux is a chronic disorder with a progressive course which involves the movement of some of the stomach acid and enzymes back up through the esophagus. This could cause inflammation and pain. The consequences can be serious and can include cancer, recurrent pneumonia, esophagitis, and bronchitis (DeVeer et al., 2008). The following are several signs and symptoms of GERD.

- Rumination (bringing food back up that has not been fully digested and re-chewing it)
- Difficulty gaining weight
- Vomiting
- Vomiting of blood (hematemesis)
- Iron deficiency anemia
- Sinus inflammation
- Excessive saliva
- Pharyngitis
- Sore throat
- Complaints of tightness in the chest or chest pain
- Coughing
- Difficulty breathing

The treatments for GERD usually include introducing dietary changes, such as an anti-reflux diet, and avoiding substances that can stimulate the stomach to produce greater amounts of acid. In addition, elevating the head of the bed can help with nighttime symptoms. Antacids are also often part of the treatment plan.

Constipation. Individuals at high risk for constipation include those with limited mobility, those with poor fluid intake, those on multiple medications, especially psychotropic and anticonvulsant medications, or those with syndromes with lower GI difficulties.

2. **Urological Conditions.** There are a number of urological conditions that can be associated with an intellectual disability. For example, individuals with Down syndrome are at an increased risk for obstruction of the lower urinary track and renal hypoplasia

(Bosch, 2003). The side effects of the long term use of psychotropic medications used to treat psychiatric conditions or behavioral challenges can include neurogenic bladders. Also, some individuals with an intellectual disability may have small bladders and/or poor bladder tone which can result in difficulties with urinary incontinence (Bosch, 2003) and increase the risk for urinary infections. If an individual has quadriplegia, the person may also be at risk for urinary tract infections. If recurring urinary tract infections are noted among males with an intellectual disability, it is important to rule out prostate problems.

3. **Asthma.** In our experience, asthmatic conditions have often gone undetected among this population. Shortness of breath and tightness in the chest can cause severe anxiety. Asthma can also lead to fatigue and irritability.

The following are some early warning signs of asthma (http://my.clevelandclinic.org):

- Frequent coughing, particularly at night
- Daytime fatigue and irritability
- Signs of a cold, allergies, or upper respiratory infections (including a headache or runny nose or sore throat)
- Feelings of restlessness
- Itchy, watery, or glassy eyes
- Difficulties sleeping
- Tightness in the chest
- Wheezing

4. **Sleep apnea.** Sleep apnea is a sleep disorder in which an individual's breathing is interrupted during sleep. There are pauses in breathing throughout the night. There are three types of sleep apnea including central, obstructive, or mixed, which is a combination of the obstructive and central forms (Vgontzas & Kales, 1999). Untreated, this can result in daytime fatigue and sleepiness. Some individuals can even present with symptoms simulating depression. The diagnosis of sleep apnea is made by an overnight sleep study called a polysomnogram. It is important to note that individual's with Down syndrome are particularly at risk for this condition (Stray-Gundersen, 1995).

5. **Seizures.** Seizure disorders occur with greater frequency among individuals with an intellectual disability, with a prevalence rate of 21% versus 1% for the general population (Nugent, 1997).

There are basically two types of seizures: generalized and partial. The type of seizure refers to how much of the brain is involved in, or is experiencing, abnormal electrical activity. The form, intensity, and duration of the seizures are related to the number and type of brain cells that are affected.

The following is a brief summary of the different types of seizures:

a. *Generalized seizures*. In this type of seizure the entire brain is affected. The individual experiences unconsciousness and convulsions, such as in tonic-clonic seizures.

b. *Partial seizures*. In partial seizures, there is abnormal electrical activity occurring in a part of the brain. Included in this category are complex partial seizures, which have also been known as psychomotor seizures or temporal lobe epilepsy. These are brief, episodic changes which are associated with changes in the person's behavior and mental status.

Pseudoseizures. Various terms have been used in describing pseudoseizures. They have also been classified as psychogenic seizures or nonepileptic seizures (PNES). They are events that resemble seizures and may be misdiagnosed as seizures, but they are considered psychological in nature or origin. According to Benbadis, and Heriaud (2002), psychogenic non-epileptic seizures are not the result of a physical abnormality but they can be a reaction to stress, trauma, and strong emotions, and they are usually involuntary. They can also be the result of faking or feigning, in which case they are then considered voluntary. They can be difficult to diagnose because they may co-exist with a genuine seizure disorder, and they can resemble epileptic seizures. However, they are not associated with abnormal cortical electrical charges (DeLeon, Uy, & Gutshall, 2005). De Leon et al. (2005) described behaviors characteristic of pseudoseizures as unresponsive staring, minor motor movements, bizarre behaviors, and generalized movements.

Medical Causes of Specific Psychiatric Symptoms

In determining whether or not a medical condition can account for specific psychiatric symptoms, it is important to ensure that the individual has had a thorough medical examination. It is also important to consider well documented associations between certain medical conditions and certain psychiatric disorders. For example, 50% of individuals with Parkinson's disease may experience a major depressive episode at some point during the course of their illness (First & Tasman, 2004). It is also very important to consider the possibility of any CNS (central nervous system) manifestations of specific syndromes which caused the intellectual disability. For example, for someone who has Fragile X syndrome, hyperactivity is usually present.

The following is a list of some more common medical contributors to or causes of depression among both the general population and among individuals with an intellectual disability:

1. **Endocrine disorders**. Thyroid conditions, including hyperthyroidism or hypothyroidism, can present as psychiatric disorders. Both hyperthyroidism and hypothyroidism can cause variable moods and symptoms of anxiety. Hypoglycemia should also be considered as it can impact mood.

2. **Nutritional deficiencies.** Deficiencies in Vitamin B-1 (thiamine), Vitamin B-2 (Riboflavin), B-6 (Pyridoxine), B-12, and folate, along with possible iron deficiencies should be ruled out. Deficiencies in calcium are also important to rule out. For example, hypocalcemia can result in fatigue, depression, and emotional lability.

3. **Neurological disorder.** Conditions such as multiple sclerosis, Parkinson's disease and Alzheimer's dementia can result can result in depression.

4. **Cancer.** Cancers, including lung cancer and pancreatic cancer, can contribute to, or cause, depression.

5. **Cardiovascular disease.** Strokes, heart attacks, cardiomyopathy, and congestive heart failure are all cardiac conditions that can contribute to, or result in, depression.

Review of Systems

A review of medical systems can be helpful in identifying underlying physical illnesses.

If changes or abnormalities are noted in any of the following categories, further medical evaluations may be warranted:

1. **Sensory.** Have there been any changes in hearing or vision?

2. **Oral Health.** Does the individual present with any signs of dental problems such as a toothache, verbal reports of pain, a decreased appetite, changes in chewing, agitation, hand-biting, or self-injurious behavior localized to areas of the face? Are the gums healthy or do they bleed? Does the person have bad breath unrelated to teeth brushing?

3. **Cardiovascular.** Is edema present? Does the individual fatigue easily? How is the individual's peripheral circulation?

4. **Skin.** How is the integrity of the skin? Are there rashes, bruises, or wounds present? Is the individual scratching or itching?

5. **Gastrointestinal.** Have there been any changes in the individual's elimination pattern? Have there been any incidents of

nausea or vomiting? Have there been any alterations in the nutritional status or any difficulties swallowing?

    6. **Genitourinary.** It is important to assess for any of the following:
- Distention/retention
- Bladder incontinence in someone previously continent
- Burning/dysuria
- Vaginal discharge
- Urethral discharge
- Urinary frequency or urgency
- Changes in menses, including heavy or absent periods

    7. **Neurological System.** Does the individual have headaches, tremors, seizures, incidents of fainting, or changes in level of consciousness?

    8. **Respiratory.** Is the individual experiencing any shortness of breath, wheezing, cough, sinus congestion, or sleep apnea?

    9. **Musculoskeletal.** How is the person's balance and gait? Does the individual have arthritis, scoliosis, or contractures?

Pain Assessments

It is important to not overlook or underestimate the effect that chronic pain can have on someone's behavior or psychiatric condition. Consequently, it is very important to assess for any pain the individual may be experiencing. There appears to be a hesitancy sometimes on the part of care providers to ask an individual if he or she is in pain. Care providers may be reluctant to ask because they believe the individual is attention-seeking and the answers will not be valid. They may believe the individual will falsely answer "yes" to the question in order to solicit more attention. Even so, it is important to ask and to observe for any pain-related behaviors.

Zwakhalen, Van Dongen, Hamers, and Abu-Sadd (2004) conducted a study of nurses who were providing care to individuals with an intellectual disability. They found that the nurses identified the following signs as common indicators of pain: facial expressions, moving in unusual ways, not using a part of their body, and various vocalizations, including moaning and crying.

When assessing for pain, it is important be aware of the individual's current medical conditions and whether or not those conditions are progressive and can result in pain or increased pain levels. Pain can contribute to, or even result in, depression as well as sleep disturbances. Therefore, it is important to obtain information regarding the individual's sleeping habits and to identify any changes in sleeping habits. In assessing for pain, it is also important to observe changes in ambulation including dropping to the ground (which can be mislabeled as non-compliance) and sitting in odd postures. Also, look for changes in the individual's affect around certain activities. For example, does the person become irritable when asked to participate in certain activities?

Interventions for addressing pain. When working with a person who is suspected to be experiencing pain, it is important to provide the following interventions:

1. Advocate for the individual and ensure proper medical follow-up so that the condition causing the pain is treated. This may involve a referral to a pain management specialist or clinic.

2. Ensure pain medications are included in the treatment plan, if needed.

3. Develop an individualized protocol to treat or manage the pain. This may include the introduction of a daily exercise routine, the application of cold compresses to an area, or ensuring the individual has periods of rest throughout the day, etc.

Barriers to Health Care for Individuals with an Intellectual Disability

There are a variety of challenges to obtaining the proper health care for individuals with an intellectual disability. This includes a shortage of physicians and other medical care professionals who are trained in the complicated health care needs of this population. The complexity of issues can result in consultations requiring more time from professionals without increased financial compensation for the medical providers.

Obtaining cooperation from the person for medical appointments or tests can be an obstacle. An individual with an intellectual disability may be fearful of attending a physician's appointment or undergoing medical procedures, even if they are non-invasive procedures. Fear and anxiety may result in behavioral problems while at an appointment, such as aggressive behaviors or property destruction, etc. Resistance may necessitate a level of sedation in order to receive the appropriate medical care or evaluations. Levels of sedation have ranged from the dispensing of oral sedating medications, such as Lorazepam, to monitored anesthesia care (also referred to as MAC sedation). Mechanical restraints, such as soft tie restraints, have also been used. This leads to issues of obtaining informed consent which can be confusing. If the individual does not have a guardian, but lacks the ability to provide informed consent, identifying the person who can provide consent for them can be a time-consuming and confusing process often lacking in protocol.

Due to the potential complexities of the medical care for individuals with an intellectual disability, several doctors may be involved. There may be a team of health care professionals monitoring the individual's health status including a neurologist, psychiatrist, psychologist, etc. This requires a greater coordination of care among the treating professionals in order to avoid any redundant assessments, missed information, or contraindicated treatments. Since the individual may not be able to communicate symptoms directly, identifying underlying medical issues may require a higher level of communication among these various disciplines as specific medical rule outs are considered. This may task caretakers to do more work in obtaining the results of the consultations and bringing them to the various medical appointments and obtaining signed release forms so that the different specialists can speak to each other.

Preparing for medical appointments. When accompanying an individual with an intellectual disability to a physician's appointment, the following strategies may be helpful, particularly if the individual tends to be resistive or anxious:

- Try to make the appointments early in the day so that there is less of a likelihood of having to wait for the physician.
- Have an activity bag ready which has items that can maintain the individual's attention and provide distracting and interesting activities. Waiting in the waiting room can increase anxiety. Therefore, waiting in the car or outside the office, can decrease the likelihood of behavioral problems. Bring a cell phone and give the receptionist your cell phone number so you can be called when the doctor is ready.
- For an individual who is not toilet trained, it is important to bring a change of clothes in case of an episode of incontinence. Sources of physical discomfort may increase the likelihood of a behavioral outburst in the office.
- Ensure the individual is not hungry or thirsty, unless foods or liquids have to be restricted due to medical tests.
- Attempts to desensitize the individual's fears can be made prior to the actual appointment or evaluation. The desensitization of fears involves gradually exposing the person to the feared situation in very small increments until the fear fades.
- Provide the person with a highly preferred item or activity

following the physician's appointment to help ensure he or she experiences more positive associations with the visit.

- If it can be anticipated that the individual may be resistive, it is helpful to have another adult present. If the individual's behavior escalates to the extent that the person has to leave the office and go to the car, this will still leave one person to speak with the physician.

- Bring along a list of all of the medications for the physician. It can be helpful to have a notebook or a binder that has a section for releases, medications, medical history, reports from physicians, physicians' names, numbers, and office addresses, etc. It is too easy to forget important information when you are trying to deal with behavioral challenges.

It is also helpful in preparing for medical appointments to bring a complete list of all the medications the individual is taking. Since several different physicians with different specialties may be involved, it is important that they know what medications may have been added or deleted by other physicians. It is also important to ensure that the caretakers who are escorting the individual are knowledgeable about the issues that need the doctor's attention. All too often someone may be escorting the person with the intellectual disability who has little knowledge of the description, extent, or duration of the symptoms, or even the person's medical history. The quality of the medical consultation is impacted by the quality of the information being provided to the physician.

Pharmacological Treatments

Due to the use of psychotropic medications among individuals with an intellectual disability and psychiatric disorders, the following section provides a brief overview of their uses, rationale, and potential side effects.

Rationale for the use of psychotropic medications. Psychotropic medications are used to treat mental disorders with the goal of improving an individual's life. The word "psychotropic" is derived from the Greek language where "psyche" refers to the mind and "tropic" means to tend to change or alter. Therefore, psychotropic medications are meant to alter the mind. They are used to address abnormalities in mood or abnormal thought processes. Among the general population, they are used to treat symptoms related to anxiety disorders, depressive disorders, and psychotic disorders. Although they may be used to treat these disorders among individuals with an intellectual disability, they can also be used to address specific behaviors. The primary use is to address a specific set of symptoms associated with a disorder. The secondary use is to utilize the side effects of a medication to address the symptom. For example, anti-seizure and antipsychotic medications can be used to address aggressive behaviors because the side effects are calming.

Prerequisites for the use of psychotropic medications. Psychotropic medications should be used as a part of an overall treatment plan. The treatment plan should be derived from a comprehensive bio-psychosocial assessment which considers all aspects of the individual's life. According to First and Tasman (2004), the following are suggested prerequisites for the use of psychotropic medications:

1. A psychiatric evaluation should be conducted to identify any existing psychiatric conditions, and the psychotropic medication should correspond to the conditions.

2. A comprehensive medical evaluation should be conducted to ensure that all medical rule outs contributing to, or causing, the symptoms have been considered and addressed.

3. In the cases that a psychiatric disorder has not been identified, there should be a comprehensive treatment plan that includes evidence that all less-intrusive interventions have been attempted and have not been successful. If a psychiatric disorder has been identified, the degree to which the psychiatric symptoms are negatively impacting the person's life should be assessed in order to determine if medications are necessary.

4. A reliable data collection system should be introduced to measure the symptoms believed to reflect a psychiatric disorder. There should also be a functional analysis conducted which identifies the antecedent conditions and the consequences of the individual's behaviors.

5. The appropriate consents should be obtained prior to the administration of the medications.

A target-symptom approach to prescribing psychotropic medications. There are some circumstances in which a target-symptom approach to the use of psychotropic medications is warranted. These are situations in which the person is exhibiting severe behaviors and the behaviors are significantly interfering with the quality of the individual's life. In these instances, the medication is based on a specific behavioral-pharmacological hypothesis rather than on a specific psychiatric condition. Even so, psychotropic medications should not be used solely to suppress a problematic behavior without considering the impact it can have on the individual's functioning level and overall quality of life. The administration of psychotropic medications should not be the only treatment objective.

Since it becomes more difficult to make specific and reliable psychiatric diagnoses among individuals whose cognitive functioning levels are within the severe and profound ranges, clinicians may need to focus on one or more behavioral symptoms as the targets of treatment. According to King (2006), "Even when a specific diagnosis can be made with confidence the clinician should also assess for behavioral symptoms that may be appropriate targets of treatment." King (2006) identified the following behavioral challenges as potential targets of pharmacological and/or behavioral treatment in the context of a *DSM-IV-TR* diagnosis, or on their own if the clinician is unable to identify a specific diagnosis:

- Self-injurious behavior
- Aggression
- Hyperactivity and impulsivity
- Social withdrawal

Side effects of psychotropic medications. All psychotropic medications have potential side effects. The effects of these medications on individuals with an intellectual disability may not be the same as those experienced by the general population. As Levitas (1997) noted, with an intellectual disability the impact of the medications on the brain are not always known because the brain functioning has already been compromised. Therefore, it may require different medication trials, and it is important to keep data regarding the changes in behavior and any new behaviors that may reflect side effects. In addition, after beginning a medication there is an adjustment period. The individual may also develop such adverse side effects that the medication may need to be discontinued. Side effects are more likely to occur when medications are started or when the dosages are increased. It is helpful to implement medication time lines and review the frequencies of behaviors relative to the initiation and changes in dosages of medications. This can also help to detect behaviors that are indicative of medication side effects.

Multiple psychotropic medication use. The use of multiple psychotropic medications as part of a medication regimen has become more common in treating both the general psychiatric population as well as individuals with an intellectual disability and psychiatric disorders. There are two types of multiple drug use:

1. *Combination treatment.* This involves the use of two or more drugs to treat specific clusters of symptoms and/or diagnoses.

2. *Augmentation treatment.* This involves the addition of one or more drugs to the existing drug in order to increase the effectiveness of the primary medication.

The following general principles of multiple medication use is taken from the *Standards for Multiple Drug Use (DMR Medical Advisory)* prepared by Dr. Robert S. White (1998):

1. Target symptoms should be clearly defined, and the medication should be indicated for at least one of the diagnoses or for the symptom cluster.

2. It most cases, it is recommended to begin with one drug and select the medication that is likely to produce the least side effects. The effectiveness of the medication should be assessed before adding more medications.

3. It is important to define the target symptoms being addressed and to establish criteria for success or failure. The starting dose and maximum dose should be identified along with the length of the medication trial.

4. If there is a treatment failure, the medication should be discontinued and consideration given to introducing a new medication.

5. If only a partial response to the medication is achieved, consider augmenting it with one or more augmenting medications. This could include a drug of a different class or one of the same class.

6. If the primary drug successfully treats a symptom cluster but leaves other symptom clusters untreated, consider combination treatment. Combination usually includes a drug from a different class.

7. It is recommended that only one medication be added at a time in order to determine its effectiveness. If too many medications are added at once, it can be difficult to determine the effectiveness of each drug.

8. Before a drug is considered to be ineffective, it should be given at an adequate dose for an adequate amount of time.

9. There should be ongoing monitoring for medication side effects and drug interactions.

10. The use of the medications should be evaluated regularly and the dosage should be lowered or discontinued whenever possible. Monitor carefully for side effects and drug-drug interactions.

Chapter 5

Identifying Diagnoses and Formulating Intervention Plans

When working with people who have such complex behavioral, medical, and psychological profiles, it can be difficult to decide where to focus treatment. This chapter will provide guidelines to identify and rule out specific areas of focus. It is understood that many of the readers may not be involved in conducting the assessment; however, input from care providers about these areas is critical. Therefore, it is important to be knowledgeable about the information that is being gathered. Obtaining information across a variety of areas in the life of a person, and from a variety of sources, may provide clues. The information obtained from these areas can help to identify not only psychiatric disorders but it can also help to identify other causes of behavioral challenges, such as medical conditions. The information can then be used to develop intervention plans.

Exploring the biological, social, and psychological factors that influence behavior is critical to understanding all of the forces which can impact the life of a person with a dual diagnosis. Gathering information in numerous areas of the person's life can help to ensure that the assessment process is comprehensive and there is a deeper understanding of the person. A variety of clinical disciplines may be involved in this process, including nursing, psychiatry, social work, psychology, and speech therapy. The following are suggested categories to explore and questions to consider in trying to understand the whole person and determine if a psychiatric condition is present.

Developmental History

Obtaining a developmental history can be important in discovering the cause of the intellectual disability. Was it the result of a head injury or of a genetic disorder? Did the individual suffer a stroke as a child? Was the cause of the intellectual disability ever identified? This information may be important in determining whether some of the behavioral challenges or psychiatric symptoms can be linked to the events which caused the intellectual disability. This can have implications for treatment strategies and behavioral interventions. There are some syndromes which cause or predispose an individual to psychiatric disorders. For example, individuals with Fragile X syndrome may have higher incidence of anxiety disorders. If a syndrome caused the intellectual disability, it is also important to know if the syndrome is likely to result in deterioration in health or cognitive functioning. Therefore, the following questions are helpful to consider and typically are obtained and referenced in assessments by social workers, psychiatrists, or psychologists.

Developmental History

- As an infant and toddler, did the person reach speech and motor milestones in a typical timeframe?
- Were there delays in the individual's developmental milestones and did these delays occur after a normal period of development?
- What is the nature of the intellectual disability and was a cause ever identified?
- Is a syndrome involved? If so, are there behaviors commonly associated with the syndrome? Is there a known behavioral phenotype?
- Were there any psychiatric diagnoses given during childhood that are still present?
- Were there any childhood diseases during childhood that have current implications? For example, is the individual a pediatric stroke victim?

Medical Conditions

Individuals with an intellectual disability often have complex medical issues. These issues can impact the presence of a psychiatric disorder in many ways. First, some behavioral characteristics that accompany a medical condition can mimic a psychiatric disorder. Second, the side effects of some medication used to treat medical conditions can mimic a psychiatric disorder. Third, the increased stress of coping with a medical condition can increase the likelihood that a psychiatric disorder will develop.

The following questions are helpful to ask as part of the assessment process in order to determine the impact a medical condition may have on an individual's psychiatric symptoms, since medical conditions may cause symptoms, mimic psychiatric symptoms, or exacerbate them:

Medical Considerations

Current Medical Conditions

- What are the individual's current medical conditions?
- Is the person ambulatory and have there been any changes in ambulation? If so, has this change been gradual or has it had an acute onset?
- Does the person have an unsteady gait and a history of falls, and, if so, when was the last fall and did the person sustain a head injury?

Medication History

- Are there any allergies to medications (or allergies in general)?
- What are the individual's current medications and their dosages? Have there been any recent changes in medication, including either changes in dosages, types of medications, or medication administration times? This should include all medications, such as over-the-counter medications, herbal supplements, prescription medications, and psychotropic medications.
- Are the dosages at the appropriate level? Are the medications at therapeutic, sub-therapeutic, or toxic levels?
- Is the individual undergoing any medication titrations (i.e., scheduled decreases or increases)? If so, what are the reasons for the changes? Have these changes been introduced in the past and, if so, what was the response?

continues

— continued —

- Is there a psychotropic medication history available, including a history of the effectiveness of the medication and side effects? Also, is there a history of medication non-compliance?
- Does the individual have a history of refusing or cheeking medications? Sometimes the behaviors may be the result of the individual not taking the medications and instead hiding them.

Medical appointments
- What recent medical appointments/tests have been scheduled or conducted? What are past test results?
- Does the individual cooperate with routine medical appointments and clinics, etc.? Has this impaired the individual's ability to receive appropriate medical care?

As part of a review of medical conditions, it is also important to review weight trends, nutrition, and eating. Fluctuations in weight can be symptomatic of depressive disorders, anxiety disorders, or eating disorders. Weight change can also be a sign of an underlying medical condition. Therefore, reviewing weight histories, specifically looking for significant fluctuations in weight, can be very important. It may be one of the first signals of declining health in a non-verbal individual.

It is also important to look for any changes in the individual's motor functioning. The onset of ambulation changes can be the result of an underlying neurological condition, etc. Psychomotor retardation or agitation can be reflective of a depression or bipolar disorder.

Changes in psychotropic medications can produce behavioral changes as a result of side effects. Therefore, it is important to review the individual's current medications and whether any new behaviors correlate with the introduction or change in medications.

In addition to this information, the information obtained from a medical systems review (referenced in Chapter 4) conducted by medical personnel, is important in completing a comprehensive assessment. Typically medical personnel, such as nurses, physicians, and psychiatrists gather this information. However, psychologists may also be reviewing information obtained in these areas given the impact it can have on behavior and mental functioning.

Psychiatric History

If the individual has had previous or current psychiatric consultations, or a history of psychiatric hospitalizations, obtaining the following information can be helpful:

Psychiatric Histories

- Does the individual have a history of psychiatric diagnoses? When were these diagnoses given and are they still current? If the past diagnoses are not the same as the current ones, are there common denominators to the various diagnoses, such as frequent and significant mood changes, impulsiveness, etc.?
- Is there a family history of psychiatric issues?
- Is there a history of admissions to psychiatric hospitals? If so, what were the reasons for admission? Are there any trends or patterns to the dates of admission? Does it suggest a psychiatric condition that is more cyclical?

Reviewing any previous admission and discharge reports from psychiatric facilities can provide information regarding the course of symptoms, previous diagnostic impressions from the admitting psychiatrists, and the course of treatment while in the hospital. Usually the history and admitting physical examinations (referred to as H & P) also include toxicology screens which can be helpful in identifying individuals with substance use histories. The admission and discharge reports also have information regarding the results of mental status examinations.

If there are psychiatric diagnoses in the individual's record, caution should be applied. Sometimes a psychiatric diagnosis may be continued throughout the individual's record and history although it may not be valid. Certain diagnoses seem to be more common than others, such as Schizoaffective Disorder, Bipolar Disorder NOS, and Intermittent Explosive Disorder. Given the complexity of the evaluation process, it is important to re-evaluate these diagnoses and not assume that the psychiatric diagnosis which is carried over in the individual's record for many years is valid. If a variety of psychiatric diagnoses are present, it is helpful to look for a common denominator. For example, is mood instability an underlying symptom of the various diagnoses that have been given?

Information regarding psychiatric histories are usually compiled or referenced in consultations written by psychiatrists and psychologists, as well as noted in social service evaluations written by social workers. However, other disciplines such as nursing, rehabilitation therapists, and speech therapists may also reference psychiatric histories because the symptoms may impact so many areas of an individual's life.

Communication Skills

The level to which a person can communicate thoughts and feelings has a tremendous impact on the interpretation of the symptoms. A lack of a formal communication system may result in more behavioral challenges because the individual cannot get his or her needs met effectively which can result in increased frustration. If the person has difficulty communicating, it leaves others to make guesses. Since diagnosing psychiatric conditions relies so heavily on self-report, this makes accurately identifying psychiatric disorders much more challenging. The following questions are helpful regarding communication skills:

Communication

- What is the level of the individual's expressive language? How does the person currently express wants and needs? Does this occur through verbal expressions or non-verbal means such as gesturing or leading others to the desired objects or activities?
- What is the individual's receptive language skill level? Can the person follow basic verbal instructions, and to what level and degree?
- Has there been any formalized testing of language abilities and if so, when was it done and what were the results?
- What is the person's ability to communicate about abstract concepts such as describing severity and duration of symptoms?
- Has there been a change in the person's communication style? If so, describe the change and length of occurrence? When did the change first appear?
- Does the individual have hearing deficits that may impact communicative abilities?

Assessing the type of communication pattern the individual has and whether or not there have been changes, provides clues as to whether there may be an underlying psychiatric or medical condition. For example, does the individual engage in prolonged vocalizations that could be suggestive of a manic episode? This may be the equivalent of pressured and more rapid speech in an individual who is verbal. If the individual used to talk but has lost that ability, could it be the result of a dementia or a trauma-based reaction? If the person is not talking as much, this may suggest a depressive disorder and reflect social withdrawal which can occur with depression. Consequently, looking for changes in the pattern, rate, fluency, and type of communication are important. Psychologists, clinical social workers, and psychiatrists reference information regarding speech in their evaluations as part of their mental status examinations and observations of an individual.

Behavioral Challenges

Often a psychiatric condition is considered because a person presents with an unusual or challenging behavior pattern. It is important to obtain a detailed description of the challenging behaviors which is often done by a psychologist or a behavior analyst. This becomes particularly important in order to ensure that the behavior is well described and defined. Behaviors that reflect changes in energy level, changes in sleep, a dysregulation of mood, disturbances of thought or perception, and changes in cognitive abilities may signal the presence of a psychiatric disorder. Individuals with psychiatric disorders may exhibit more aberrant or unusual behaviors. When trying to determine if the behavioral pattern is the result of an underlying psychiatric condition, the following questions may be helpful:

Behavioral Challenges

- Does the individual have any current behavioral challenges? If so, what are they? This should include a description of the behavior in specific terms. For example, aggression can be described more specifically as incidents of kicking and punching.
- Are these behavioral challenges new?
- How long have these behaviors been occurring? What are the histories of the behaviors? When did the individual start exhibiting the behaviors?

— continues —

— continued —

- If these behaviors have not been exhibited for awhile, when did they start to re-emerge?
- What are the current frequencies of the behaviors and how severe are they?
- Have there been recent changes in either the severities or frequencies of the behaviors? Have these changes been gradual in nature or more sudden?
- Have these behaviors ever been the focus of treatment and, if so, what type of treatment? How long was the treatment provided?
- What interventions, including proactive and reactive strategies, have been used to address the behavioral challenges? Have any of these interventions been effective?
- What are the triggers for these behaviors? Is it difficult to identify triggers?
- Does the individual currently have a psychiatric diagnosis and is it consistent with the current symptoms and behavioral presentation?
- Have there been any changes in the individual's energy level, sleep patterns, affect, or level of alertness?
- Do the behaviors occur in all settings?
- Are there environments in which the behaviors do not occur?
- Do the behaviors only occur with specific individuals?
- Are there any time trends or patterns to the occurrence of the behaviors? For example, does the person exhibit the behaviors early in the morning or only in the evenings?
- Is the person engaging in any purposeful self-harm, e.g., hitting or cutting himself or herself?

The functional analysis also becomes part of the assessment of the behavioral challenges, since it helps to identify the following:

- Where does the behavior occur?
- With whom does it occur?
- In what settings does it occur?
- When does it occur?
- What is the outcome following its occurrence?

Behaviors that are the result of psychiatric conditions usually occur across settings and in the presence of a variety of individuals. The behaviors may sometimes occur without any environmental triggers. In addition, the individual does not seem to have control over the behaviors. If behavioral interventions are largely ineffective or not effective at all, it may be because the behaviors are the result of a psychiatric condition. Unusual, rapid, and significant changes in behavior can also serve as a signal of an underlying psychiatric issue. However, if there is a rapid onset of behavioral challenges, accompanied by a change in the individual's cognitive functioning, it may signal a condition triggered by an underlying medical cause rather than a psychiatric condition. If an individual has not exhibited a particular challenging behavior for a long time and it begins to re-emerge, it can be the result of stress. Stress induced behavioral regressions can result in the re-emergence of old problem behaviors that were part of the individual's repertoire months ago, or even years ago.

Self-Help Skills

Obtaining information on the individual's current level of independence with regard to daily activities of living can provide clues to the presence of psychiatric conditions. For example, it is important to look for any deterioration in the individual's abilities. It is also important to note whether or not the loss of skills or regression in skills has been gradual or sudden in onset. Regression in self-help skills, such as showering, grooming, and dressing, can occur as a result of psychiatric issues such as depression, psychosis, or dementia. Changes may also occur in response to a traumatic event such as physical or emotional abuse by a care provider. Uncontrolled seizure activity can also result in a loss of skills.

Deteriorations in skill levels can also occur as a result of learned behaviors. For example, an individual may have learned to become dependent upon others to complete the tasks of daily living. If the person takes a long time to complete a self-care task such as tooth brushing, a care provider may perform the task for the person in the interest of time. Consequently, the person becomes more dependent upon others and less self-reliant. This is reflective of a learning process rather than a psychiatric disorder. Also, obtain information regarding the person's level of cooperation with care providers during self-help tasks, specifically noting if there have been any changes in this area. Some people who have been the victims of abuse, such as sexual abuse, may exhibit resistiveness while being helped with showering or toileting.

It is also informative to obtain historical information on the highest level of task independence the individual has achieved in self-help skills. This can provide a time line noting when the regression in skills began and the possible beginning of a psychiatric illness or the introduction of another factor responsible for the regression.

With regard to the specific self-help skills and areas to explore, the following questions can provide important information:

Self-Help Skills

Grooming/Bathing/ Dressing

- Does the person have any compulsive or ritualistic behaviors around dressing or grooming?
- Is the person making frequent trips to the bathroom? Are any of these trips occurring right after eating?
- Does the person spend excessive amounts of time in the bathroom?
- Does the individual come out of the bathroom having not completed the hygiene tasks or not completed them thoroughly?
- What was the highest skill level the person had achieved in ability to perform hygiene tasks?
- Has there been a deterioration in skill level?
- Has there been a change in the person's level of cooperation if assisted by others in completing self-care tasks? Has this been a sudden or gradual change?
- Does the person have less of an interest in performing the tasks?

The time an individual spends in the bathroom completing self-care skills can also provide clues as to whether or not there is an underlying psychiatric condition. For example, if an individual is suffering from Obsessive-Compulsive Disorder (OCD), problem behaviors can be seen in compulsive or ritualistic behaviors around dressing, showering, or grooming (e.g., compulsive hand washing or turning the faucets on and off). This could result in the individual spending excessive amounts of time in the bathroom.

Individuals with eating disorders may make frequent trips to the restroom to either self-induce vomiting or because of laxative use.

They may also spend time in the bathroom checking and measuring themselves to monitor weight gain.

Several other psychiatric possibilities may exist, such as Body Dysmorphic Disorder.

This may result in a person spending excessive amounts of time in the bathroom because of a preoccupation with perceived bodily flaws. An individuals who suffers with Trichotillomania (i.e., compulsive urges to pull out their hair) may also spend excessive amounts of time in the bathroom pulling out hairs on various areas of the body.

With regard to specific self-help skills, it is also important to focus on whether or not there have been any changes around toileting and elimination. This could provide information on whether a medical condition is present as well as a psychiatric issue. For example, the following questions can be informative:

Toileting
- Has there been deterioration in bowel or bladder continence?
- Is there any history of nocturnal or diurnal enuresis or encopresis (i.e., daytime or night time urine or bowel accidents)?
- Is there any history of fecal impactions?
- Is there a co-existing GI problem impacting toileting?
- Is there a current medical condition identified for constipation and, if so, is the current bowel regimen effective in addressing the condition?

If a person with established independent toileting skills starts to have urinary accidents, this could be the result of stress or it may have an underlying medical cause. Urinary tract infections can result in an increased need to urinate and may make it difficult for a person to refrain from urinating because of increased urinary urgency. Also, with the onset of diabetes (which can occur with some of the psychotropic medications), there may be increased urination. Some of the anticonvulsant medications and psychotropic medications can cause constipation, and this may result in increased time in the bathroom.

Another area of focus is eating. It is important to notice if there have been changes in the individual's ability to eat independently or if there have been any changes in behavior around mealtimes. Not only could this help signal the presence of a psychiatric issue but it can also help signal an underlying medical issue.

Changes in appetite and changes in weight can occur with depression, anxiety, or psychosis. Changes in the person's ability to eat independently or swallow can also occur with dementia, strokes, etc.

Eating

- Is the individual able feed himself or herself or has there been a change in this?
- Is there a history of appetite changes (increases or decreases)?
- Is there a history of an eating disorder?
- Does the individual display unsafe or problematic behaviors around mealtimes, such as stealing food, overstuffing his or her mouth, eating too fast or too slow, or turning his or her head away from the food when being fed, etc.?
- Is there history of excessive fluid intake (e.g., psychogenic polydypsia)?
- Has the individual had any dysphagia evaluations or swallow studies performed?
- Does the person have a history of significant weight fluctuations?
- Does the individual have any medical conditions that contribute to difficulties eating, such as reduced chewing due to structural abnormalities?

Information regarding an individual's self-help skills is usually obtained during the course of nursing assessments, evaluations by rehabilitation therapists, and social service evaluations conducted by social workers, psychologists, and psychiatrists. Nutritionists will also look at an individual's eating abilities and behaviors that impact nutritional status.

Social Relationships

Information regarding the individual's relationships and the status of current social supports can be revealing, along with any changes in social connectedness. When trying to determine if psychiatric conditions exist for individuals with an intellectual disability, it is important to consider any changes in their social support networks.

This includes family, peer, and work relationships as well as their support team (social worker, staff, doctors, etc.). It is very important to consider any sources of interpersonal stress that a person may be experiencing. For example, does the person live in a group home and is he or she encountering difficulties with a staff member? If the person doesn't know how to deal with the staff, the individual may exhibit some behavioral challenges in response to the interpersonal stress and difficulties coping with the situation. Once the individual leaves that situation, there may be a significant decrease or absence in the problem behaviors. Since many people with dual diagnoses have little control over the relationships in their lives, it is important to examine the quality of those relationships and whether or not conflicts are present. Individuals with an intellectual disability often don't choose their housemates or the care providers who will be assisting them. If stress from interpersonal conflicts lead to increases in behavioral challenges, the behaviors may be too quickly attributed to an underlying psychiatric disorder rather than a reaction to stress.

It is also important to consider any losses the individual may have encountered in his or her social support system. This may include the loss of a family member, relative, or favorite staff member. If the individual has changed residences, it is not uncommon for the person to leave behind peers who have been friends. Some behaviors or symptoms may be reactions to the sense of loss and loneliness he or she feels, or they may be unresolved and complicated grief reactions.

In trying to consider whether or not an individual with an intellectual disability has a psychiatric disorder, it is important to explore any changes in social variables including social relatedness. Changes in social relationships, including losses, conflicts with others, and decreases or increases in social activities, can occur with certain psychiatric conditions. For example, depression will sometimes result in increased irritability, social withdrawal, and a decrease in the desire to be around people. The following are some recommended questions to ask as part of the assessment process:

Social

- Does the person like to be alone? How social is the individual?
- Has there been a change in the individual's interest in being around others?
- What is the nature and extent of the person's current social support network?
- Have there been recent changes in the social network?
- Does the individual currently have contact with family members? To what degree does that contact occur and how are those relationships? What are the reasons for any lack of interactions?
- What type of peer group does the individual have? Does the person have any close friendships?
- Does the individual enjoy spending time with peers or staff?
- Is the person reaching out in unsafe ways, such as connecting with strangers on the internet?
- What is the individual's loss history? Has the person experienced the death of a family member or friend? If so, how was this information presented?
- Has there been any change in the person's level of social relatedness?

Information regarding an individual's social relationships is often obtained by a variety of clinical disciplines, including social workers and psychologists. Rehabilitation therapists also look at an individual's socialization and leisure areas.

Work/Vocational/Day Program

Information obtained about a day program or work site attendance and performance can be helpful in uncovering psychiatric issues. The work environment is often a more structured setting, with increased demands. How the person engages in this setting can provide valuable information. A decline in attendance or motivation to perform the tasks may provide insight into the person's emotional state and help to identify a possible mood disorder or issues with anxiety. For example, if the individual intermittently runs out of the workshop or runs away from the work site, panic or anxiety may be an issue. If the person is not motivated to work it could suggest an underlying depression if accompanied by other symptoms associated with depression. If the person has difficulty attending to a task for extended periods of time, it could also suggest attentional issues that may be part of an Attention Deficit Hyperactivity Disorder (ADHD). Therefore, the following questions are helpful to consider in reviewing work histories:

Work Histories

- What jobs or vocational activities has the individual participated in and is the person currently attending any work related or day program activities?
- Is attendance consistent? Does the person attend full days or half-days?
- Is attendance inconsistent due to difficulties getting up in the morning?
- How long can the person attend to a specific task? Have there been any recent changes in the individual's ability to sustain attention and attend to tasks?
- Has there been a recent decline in work performance or in attendance?
- What was the highest job held?
- How often does the person request a change in day programs or job sites?

Leisure Skills

A person's participation in leisure skills is an important area to assess when identifying a psychiatric disorder and when developing a treatment plan for someone in the general population. However, although it is equally important to consider for people with dual diagnoses, it is often overlooked. Identify whether there has been a change in the individual's motivation to engage in recreational and leisure activities. For example, if the person is refusing to attend social events that he or she used to enjoy, it may be suggestive of a variety of psychiatric disorders including depression, anxiety, psychosis, dementia, etc. If the individual has more energy than observed previously, and that energy is a significant change in the person's baseline functioning, it may be reflective of the onset of a hypomanic or manic episode.

The following questions can help identify whether a change in leisure skills may reflect an underlying psychiatric condition:

Leisure Skills

- Does the person typically engage in leisure skills independently?

- Has there been a loss of interest in favorite hobbies or leisure activities?

- Is the person exhibiting any unusual amounts of energy toward high risk activities?

- Does the person verbally talk about wanting to participate in hobbies but not follow through?

How to Obtain the Information

In working with the general population, a clinician relies heavily on the person's self-report of symptoms and experiences in order to determine if a psychiatric condition is present.

However, the clinician may be at a disadvantage if the individual lacks the expressive language skills or the cognitive abilities to label the emotions and experiences. Thus, the information from the various areas identified as part of the assessment process may need to be obtained from a variety of sources.

Interviews with the individual. If the person possesses the language skills, it is important to listen to the individual's perspective on the situation, a description of his or her symptoms, the reasons for some of the behaviors, and the individual's goals, hopes, stressors, fears, disappointments, etc. If the person is non-verbal, information can still be obtained by observing the person's body language, communication style, affect, motor skills, eye contact, level of connectedness with the people in the room, energy level, etc.

A clinician working with the general population will typically complete a mental status examination as part of the process of assessing whether or not a psychiatric condition is present. The components of a mental status examination would typically consist of obtaining information among the following categories:

- Appearance (e.g., neatly dressed or disheveled); weight
- Behavior, including motor movement
- Mood (e.g., angry, agitated)
- Affect (e.g., full range, appropriate or inappropriate, social relatedness)
- Speech (rate, volume, articulation, fluency, organization)
- Cognition (e.g., alert, lethargic)
- Orientation (time and date, name, place, and situation)
- Thought content (hallucinations, delusions, suicidal ideation or intent)
- Thought process (logical, goal directed, coherent, tangential and circumstantial)

Modifications to this typical mental status examination may be needed when working with individuals with an intellectual disability, particularly if the person is non-verbal. At the same time, it is important to assess each area. For example, if the person makes various vocalizations, has there been a change in the amount of vocalizations or the intensity? Assessing for thought content and thought processes in someone who is non-verbal is not possible among the lower levels of cognitive functioning if there is no formal speech (i.e., severe and profound intellectual disability). This is what makes it difficult to assess suicidal ideation or psychosis. For example, in order to diagnose psychosis, hallucinations and delusions need to be present. If the person cannot speak, it is very difficult to determine if he or she is hallucinating or having delusional beliefs. Therefore, the mental status examination may need to rely heavily, if not entirely on observations of the person alone and with others in different environments.

Interviews with the individual's social support network.

Interviews with collateral sources such as job coaches, residential staff, and previous care providers can be critical. The reliability of the information can increase in direct proportion to the number of people in the individual's support network who are interviewed. Sometimes, if only a few people are interviewed, there is the risk of obtaining skewed information based on their limited exposure to the person, or other factors such as burnout, etc.

If possible, it may be helpful to gain permission from the person to interview previous care providers. This can help establish what the individual's highest level of functioning has been. It can also provide more information regarding histories of the behaviors and symptom time lines.

Interviews with family members can also provide information regarding family psychiatric and medical histories. This can help to assess for a genetic predisposition to various disorders, both psychiatric and medical. Opportunities to interview family members to obtain this information is often overlooked. Interviews with family can also be invaluable in obtaining information regarding any family factors, crises, or changes in the family dynamics that may be contributing to the person's current issues or presentation. Family members can also provide a history of behavior challenges.

Review of records. Review of available records can be extremely helpful, particularly if the following information can be accessed:

- Medical evaluations including the results of any other medical specialty consultations, such as neurological or cardiology consultations
- Audiology or ophthalmology evaluations
- Any behavioral assessments (past and current), including functional analyses
- Psychological evaluations
- Psychiatric evaluations (past and current)
- Past incident reports
- Placement histories, including the types of residences the individual lived in and the reasons for moving
- Agency summaries or quarterly reports

Assessment measures. Various assessment tools can also be used to assist in the diagnostic process including several standardized assessment measures. However, these instruments should not be used as the sole basis, or even primary basis, for making a psychiatric diagnosis. They may be used as part of an overall assessment process with information obtained from numerous sources.

Below is a list of several instruments designed to assist in identifying psychiatric symptoms.

Aberrant Behavior Checklist. This instrument was originally developed to monitor the effects of psychotropic medications on behavior. However, it was later thought that the assessment measure may have a greater utility. This is a checklist completed by people who know the individual well. It was developed by Aman and Singh (1986). The responses to the checklist are then categorized according to five scales and rated in terms of their significance. The five scales are as follows: Irritability, Lethargy, Stereotypy, Hyperactivity, and Inappropriate Speech.

The Psychiatric Assessment Schedule for Adults with Developmental Disability (PAS-ADD) Checklist (Revised). This is a 25-item checklist designed as a screening tool for use when deciding whether further assessment of an individual's mental health status is warranted. It was constructed to identify a range of problems, which may be occurring as a result of a mental illness (Moss et al., 1998). It is scored on a four-point scale and it consists of a checklist of life events and symptoms. It produces scores relating to affective and psychotic disorders as well as a score related to a possible organic condition such as a dementia.

The Diagnostic Assessment for the Severely Handicapped II. This is an 84-item measure which is completed by care providers and individuals who know the person well. They rate each item, and there are 13 subscales: Anxiety, Depression, Mania, PDD/Autism, Schizophrenia, Stereotypies, Self-Injury, Elimination, Eating, Sleeping, Organic, Sexual, and Impulse Control. This is a scale with a direct link to the *DSM-IV* (Matson, 1995).

Reiss Screen for Maladaptive Behavior. Originally a 38-item scale was created by Reiss in 1986 followed by a 60-item scale in 1988. It is a questionnaire completed by people who know the person well, and it is a screening tool for mental health issues among individuals with an intellectual disability. Their responses are placed on the following nine scales: Aggressive Behavior, Autism, Psychosis, Paranoia, Depression (B), Depression (P), Dependent, Avoidant and Other Maladaptive Behavior.

The Hierarchy

Information obtained from the various areas of the person's life is used to evaluate behaviors according to a hierarchy. The hierarchy is as follows:

1. Are the behaviors the result of medical conditions?
2. Are the behaviors the result of psychiatric conditions?
3. Are the behaviors learned?

If the behaviors are not the result of medical issues, the second level of consideration is psychiatric. For example, are the behaviors the result of a specific psychiatric condition such as an anxiety disorder or a depressive disorder? If the behaviors do not seem to be the result of a medical or psychiatric condition, then the third category considered is that of a learned behavior. Learned behaviors result in some type of gain for the individual, such as attention, task avoidance, etc. It is possible that the individual's behavioral presentation is a combination of two or more of these variables. Complicating the assessment process is the fact that some behaviors may have begun in response to medical conditions or psychiatric issues, but now also have a learned element to them. For example, someone who started limping in response to pain, may now limp with greater intensity due to the amount of attention received. Therefore, what began in response to a medical cause now has a learned component.

Behavioral Crises: A Problem-Solving Perspective

Sometimes a clinician is asked to provide input and make recommendations quickly in response to a trend of escalating behaviors or behavioral crises. Sometimes the individual is on the verge of losing a residential placement because of behavioral challenges or close to receiving a discharge notice from a vocational setting or day program. In addition, the behavioral challenges may be escalating to the extent that one or more psychiatric admissions have occurred. The following is presented as a problem-solving strategy for addressing those behavioral crises or as a response to a trend of escalating behavioral challenges. Although a comprehensive evaluation should still be conducted, obtaining information among the following categories can expedite the assessment process and may lead to a quick resolution:

Obtain a history of the challenging behavior. It is important to identify whether or not these behaviors are new or existing behaviors that have increased in frequency and/or severity. If they are new behaviors, ask what has changed in the individual's life recently. Is the individual reacting to changes in the environment, to changes in routine, or to changes in the social support network? If the behavior is long-standing but has recently increased in its severity and frequency, it may be indicative of a stress induced regression. If it is a new behavior with an abrupt onset, it may be more suggestive of an underlying medical issue.

Conduct an abbreviated functional analysis. A thorough functional analysis can be a time-consuming process. The following are some ways to obtain the pertinent information in the shortest amount of time:

- Where: Where does the behavior occur and where does it not occur? If it only occurs in certain situations, it is more likely to be related to a situational stressor. If it occurs across all environments, it is more likely to be a medically or psychiatrically caused behavior. It may have started in one environment, but has carried over into other environments. Therefore, it is also helpful to find out, if possible, in what environment the behavior first occurred.

- What: What events occur just prior to the behavior? If no triggers can be identified and it occurs truly "out of the blue," it maybe internally driven and the result of a medical, psychiatric, or sensory issue.
- When: Identify any time trends surrounding the behavior. For example, is the behavior most likely to occur in the early morning? This can provide clues to possible physical states such as fatigue, changes in the environment, and staff shift changes in a facility.
- Who: Does the behavior only occur around certain people? If so, examine the nature of those interactions.

Medical systems review. Explore the possibility of an underlying medical cause that may need further medical evaluation. It is helpful to obtain information regarding the various medical systems to see if there are any changes in an area that may suggest an underlying medical issue. This would include assessing for any changes in eating, ambulation, elimination, activity level, mental alertness, motor activity, sensory changes, etc.

Consider the individual's medical history. The behaviors can be the result of a pre-existing medical condition which may have returned after a period of remission. The behaviors may also be the result of a progressive medical condition. When obtaining information about the individual's health status, it is important to avoid assumptions. Sometimes a care provider or family member may say that the individual has had recent medical evaluations with no remarkable findings. It is important to ask the nature of the tests and the evaluations that were conducted. The quality of the medical evaluation may have hinged on the information, or lack of information, provided to the physicians by the caretakers. If the information was lacking, the examination may have been a precursory one or the individual's behaviors may have posed a barrier to a medical evaluation even though the individual went to the clinic.

Medications. Assess for any recent changes in medication, including all medications, even over-the-counter medications. It can be helpful if a time line is constructed of the medications to determine whether there is any correlation between the introduction of medications, changes in dosages, and changes in behavior. Assess for any drug interactions or medication side effects. It is also important to ensure that if an individual is taking a psychotropic medication which needs periodic blood draws, the current blood panels have been done to ensure the medication is within the therapeutic range.

Illegal substances. This issue is often overlooked in individuals with an intellectual disability, but it is important to assess for any illegal substance use. If the individual has had a recent psychiatric hospitalization, a toxicology screen may have been done which can assist in identifying any illegal substance use. The possibility of substance abuse should not only be considered for individuals with a mild to moderate intellectual disability but also for individuals who are functioning cognitively within the lower ranges. Unfortunately, there have been situations in which illegal drugs have been given to individuals with an intellectual disability by those asked to provide for their care.

Psychiatric diagnosis. Obtain information about whether or not the individual has a psychiatric diagnosis or has had one in the past that could account for some of the current behavioral challenges. Reviewing the record for information regarding diagnoses (both past and present) can be very helpful. The current behavioral issues may be manifestations of a psychiatric disorder that has recently been exacerbated or is no longer in remission. It is important to also consider commonly occurring co-morbid psychiatric diagnoses. For example, if someone is depressed it is important to assess for the presence of anxiety. Where there is one anxiety disorder, it is not uncommon to have another. Individuals with Attention Deficit Disorder can also be at higher risk for anxiety disorders, etc.

Be aware of a syndrome. Be aware of any identified cause of the intellectual disability. Sometimes the intellectual disability is caused by a syndrome and there may be psychiatric, medical, and behavioral associations with the syndrome that can be influencing behavior. For example, individuals with Down syndrome have a higher rate of obstructive sleep apnea (Stray-Gundersen, 1995). This could lead to chronic daily fatigue because they are not experiencing a good night's sleep. This can produce daytime fatigue. The fatigue can lead to a lack of interest in activities, withdrawal, excessive sleeping during the day, etc., that can be misconstrued as willful and purposeful behavior or even mislabeled as depression. There may also be a behavioral phenotype, or set of behavioral characteristics that are biologically associated with a disorder. Behavioral phenotypes of genetic disorders are discussed in detail in Chapter 3 of the *DM-ID* (Levitas, Dykens, Finucane, & Kates, 2007a, 2007b).

Sleep. The impact that a lack of sleep or a disruptive sleep pattern can have on daily functioning should not be underestimated. It is important to assess for whether or not there have been any disruptions in the individual's sleep pattern. Is the individual sleeping less or sleeping more? This can provide clues to the possibility of an underlying psychiatric disorder such as an anxiety disorder or a mood disorder. Does the individual exhibit any odd behaviors during sleep? This can even provide clues to the possibility of an underlying medical condition, e.g., restless leg syndrome or sleep apnea.

Assess for adjustment or stress related reactions. Obtain information regarding whether or not there have been any recent changes in the individual's life. This could extend to changes in the job or workshop, changes in living arrangements or the living environment, as well as changes in social support and interpersonal relationships. The behavioral challenges being exhibited may be the result of stress reactions or adjustment reactions that the individual is experiencing.

Assess for a trauma history. Is there a history of known incidents of abuse that the individual has experienced? This can result in anxiety or challenging behaviors if the person is experiencing flashbacks of any traumatic events. Events or people in the individual's current environment can be reminding them of past abusive incidents or previous abusers. It is also important to consider any life situations that may have proven to be traumatic for the individual but did not necessarily involve any type of abuse.

Assess for head trauma. It is also important to assess for the possibility of a head trauma. Is there a history of a traumatic brain injury? If so, what was the nature of the injury, and were there any long-term effects? There can be behavioral disturbances that accompany traumatic brain injuries. Identifying the location and nature of the injury can help provide a greater understanding of how the injury may impact behaviors. In addition, note whether or not the behavioral disturbances were present to any degree prior to the injury.

Summary

This chapter provided many things to consider when identifying diagnoses and goals for treatment. The amount of information can be overwhelming. No single person can assess the impact of every area; however, each person on the support team should be vigilant to ensuring that each factor is considered by the appropriate person. It is important not to assume all of the medical factors are considered by the doctors and all of the behavioral and self-help factors are considered by home support people. If everyone takes the responsibility to review each component, it is more likely that a comprehensive plan will be developed.

Chapter 6

Positive Behavioral Supports

When a person with an intellectual disability presents with a challenging behavior pattern, one of the most common approaches is to identify a "behavior plan" to address that issue. Prior to the 1980's, behavioral approaches focused on the Stimulus-Response model (S-R Model) (Chaplin & Krawiec, 1974). A stimulus was identified that provoked a specific response. For example, a person screams (stimulus) and gets attention (response). This led to various contingency management interventions to address challenging behaviors. For example, a person screams (stimulus) and is ignored (response), which evolves into the person asking for help (stimulus), thus, not screaming, and getting a reward (response). Another example is a person uses a picture to communicate (stimulus) and receives a reward (response). Over the years, behavioristic approaches have evolved to include more of an S-O-R model. The "O" represents the "organism" or the individual. This includes the person's desires, wants, likes, and dislikes. Positive approaches to behavioral change are now considering the "whole person." They involve a multi-disciplinary approach to assessing the complex needs of persons with an intellectual disability. People from the individual's support groups come together to help him or her communicate personal goals and wishes.

Currently, the emphasis is on "positive behavioral support." Rather than the simplistic focus on eliminating a behavior, the goal is to understand the purpose of the behavior and why it is occurring. Positive Behavioral Support Plans focus on identifying the person's desires and identifying positive ways for them to meet those needs. Behavior management, education, and social support are combined to create or frame environments that allow people to succeed.

Behavioral Assessment and Functional Analysis

A behavioral assessment is an analysis aimed at identifying the history, presentation, purpose, and outcome of a particular behavior. The behavioral assessment aids in understanding the person and is usually conducted by a psychologist or a behavior analyst. The functional analysis is one part of the behavioral assessment. The functional analysis focuses on the cause and outcome of the behavior. It is used to identify why a person may be exhibiting a behavior, what needs are being met by the behavior, and what interventions have been effective or ineffective.

A behavioral assessment should include the following:

- Observations of the individual in various environments
- A history of the challenging behaviors, including the identified target behavior
- Specific definitions of challenging behaviors
- Interventions that have been attempted and the effectiveness of those interventions
- Outcome of the behavior (how did others respond, etc.)
- Hypotheses about the purpose of the target behavior
- A method of data collection in order to measure and record the target behavior

The Role of the Functional Analysis

A functional analysis is a systematic way to assess a person's behavior with the goal of understanding why it occurs. It serves as the foundation for the behavior plan. The approach of conducting a functional analysis was first introduced in an article by Iwata, Dorsey, Siflher, Bauman, and Richman (1982). It assumes that all behaviors occur for reasons and have meaning. A functional assessment approach assumes that behaviors do not occur without specific antecedents or triggers, even if those triggers are not always observable by others. Completing a functional analysis is even more important when the causes of the behavior are difficult to identify. For example, if the behavior has a physiological cause or the person has poor communication skills, it is often more difficult to identify the function of the behavior, necessitating an even more objective information gathering approach.

A functional assessment is more systematic than a behavior assessment, but many factors overlap. A functional assessment involves the following steps:

- Identification of the target behavior
- Data collection
- Hypothesis generation
- Plan development
- Plan implementation
- Data collection
- Review of plan effectiveness

Identification of the target behavior. When identifying a target behavior it is very important to have a clear definition of the specific behavior being addressed. The definition needs to be concrete, objective, and measurable. General terms can be confusing and lead to inaccurate data collection. For example, the term *aggression* is commonly used as a target behavior, although, it is a general term that can mean different things for different people. It is important to use specific definitions that are agreed upon by those who are documenting the behavior. The degree of specificity will depend on the individual and the variation of his or her behavior patterns. For example, the term *aggression* should be differentiated between 1) physical aggression, 2) verbal aggression, 3) property destruction, or 4) throwing items at someone. To further clarify the target behavior verbal aggression and property destruction can be more distinct.

Throwing objects at someone ← PROPERTY DESTRUCTION → Breaking property

Threats to harm ←VERBAL AGGRESSION → Cursing and yelling

Data collection. Data is collected to help identify the frequency, duration, and intensity of the behavior as well as the situation, times, and environmental factors which may be influencing the behavior. This will enable the support team to better understand the reason a behavior occurs as well as better predict high risk times. In addition, data provides a baseline. The baseline is the starting point from which to improve. If a person has a baseline of 10 incidents of physical aggression per month, a decrease in that number shows improvement, while an increase in that number shows further problems. Without the baseline number, small changes can go unnoticed. For example, a decrease from 10 incidents to 7 incidents per month is a 30% improvement. It still may appear like a lot of incidents, but it is an indication that the interventions are working.

There are several different types of data collection systems. They vary in the amount of time it takes to complete them, the type of information that is gathered, and the usefulness in tracking individual behavior patterns. For target behaviors that are infrequent, or for settings that allow time for detailed documentation, narrative recording or "ABC" Charts may be effective.

Narrative recording involves keeping a running log or narrative of the behavior as it progresses. Information can then be ordered into a sequential analysis involving the identification of the antecedents, a description of the behavior itself, and the consequences occurring as a result of the behavior (the ABC sequence). This type of data collection is most useful in the early stages of trying to identify important variables which may be triggering the behavior and maintaining it. At the same time, this does not provide quantitative data, and it can be time-consuming.

For settings in which one-on-one attention is available interval recording, frequency/event recording, or duration recording may be effective. **Interval recording** is most often used in educational settings and is a logistically difficult method of recording data. The observation period is divided into equal time intervals, such as one minute or ten minute intervals. The observer notes whether or not the behavior occurs at any time during that interval. With this method, neither frequency nor duration is measured. It measures only the occurrence or non-occurrence of the behavior. For example, how many times did a student initiate peer interaction during a ten minute interval over a sixty minute period? This data collection procedure requires continual observation throughout the interval.

Frequency/event recording is when the observer documents the number of times the behavior occurs during a specific period of time. That time period may consist of a minute, hour, etc. The behavior must have a clearly defined beginning and end point, and the frequency must be low enough to count. For example, the number of times a person makes eye contact during a one minute interval or the number of times a person asks a repetitive question during a ten minute interval. **Duration recording** is used when the observer is interested in specific aspects of the behavior. The total length of time that the behavior occurs is measured. For example, the duration a person remains seated in a chair or the length of time a person is engaged in self-stimulatory behavior is recorded.

Scatter plots can be a quick way to identify whether there is a pattern with the time of day that a target behavior is more likely to occur. It is a graph in which one axis of the graph has the time of day and the other axis has the specific day. The observer simply places a mark in the box corresponding to the day and time of day the behavior occurred. If a behavior occurs consistently at a particular time of day, it is easily identified with this type of graph. This can be very useful if there are various staff members working with the person each day.

Time sampling is the least reliable method of data collection, but the easiest. Data is collected at specified periods of time. For example, the observer notes whether or not the behavior occurs at each ten minute mark, but not how many times it occurs between those intervals. This is useful when it is difficult to do continuous recording. It is an easy and unobtrusive method that is used for very high frequency behaviors (self-stimulatory behavior). On the other hand, it is not an accurate measure of overall frequency.

When deciding which data recording system to use it is important to consider the frequency of the behavior, whether it is continuous or prompted by a specific antecedent, whether someone is required to intervene when it happens, and, most importantly, what the observer is logistically able to do. Time sampling, interval recording, frequency/event recording, and duration recording are more feasible when there is the capability for individual attention to be given to the person, such as supplemental (one-on-one) staff availability. This is often only available in specialized clinic, school, and hospital settings. Logistically, it is difficult to complete this type of recording in most group home and day program settings.

Realistically, most often the "observer" is a support person at a group home, work setting, day program, or hospital. That person is likely to have other duties that don't include documenting behavior patterns to the detail some of these systems require. It is very important to be understanding of this. There are often valid reasons a staff person does not keep accurate data. These may include:

- It is difficult to stop and write when the support staff is dealing with a high intensity behavior.

- The day is often very busy and there is no time to document during the regular hours.
- The systems that are put in place look good on paper, but can be very confusing for staff.
- When the systems are complicated the staff often don't do them, and they don't let others know they are confused.
- If the support person sees documentation as extra work that is not useful to him or her, he or she is more likely to complete it inconsistently.

Staff support is necessary when requesting documentation for many reasons, most importantly, to collect accurate data. Staff need support in developing the system, learning how to use it, and knowing what to document. If documentation is not done consistently it can lead to misleading results, which is frustrating for the staff and the person the staff are working with. Make the systems easy for the people using them. Remember, less and consistent information is better than more and inconsistent information. Also, only ask the staff to do what they believe they can do. Otherwise you may get resistance, which can lead to inaccurate data. See Appendix E for a sample data form that was developed with the input of direct care staff.

Generation of hypotheses. After the data is gathered, a hypothesis is formulated regarding the possible function of the behavior. When looking at the data, the antecedents are examined. The **antecedents** are the factors that precede the behavior. They are things that may cause the individual to become agitated, anxious, or angry or to react with the target behavior. Examples of antecedents include being asked to do something the individual does not like to do (shower, go to work, etc.), a tone of voice, interactions with a person that are negative, discussion about a person from the past that makes the individual sad, a time of day, shift change, unstructured time, etc.

Once the antecedents are identified, the next step is to identify what "need" is being met by the behavior. The need may be emotional, physical, or behavioral. Some **emotional needs** include gaining the comfort of the staff when they are feeling anxious, behavioral limits to help them feel in control when angry, an outlet for emotional energy, and bringing others to them which provides an emotional connection. It does not matter that the behavior is not socially acceptable to those around them if it is meeting their need.

Many times it is difficult for individuals with an intellectual disability to verbalize physical symptoms, therefore, the target behavior may be in response to a physical need. **Physical needs** include communicating agitation in response to physical symptoms such as physical pain, discomfort, fatigue, low blood sugar, hunger, feeling cold or hot, feeling side effects of medication, etc. **Behavioral needs** are those that change the behavioral expectation others have of them, such as gaining attention so they are not alone, avoidance of an activity they don't like, having others do a challenging task for them, social engagement, humor, and wanting to decrease independence.

The *Reiss Profile of Fundamental Goals and Motivation Sensitivities for Persons with Mental Retardation* (2001) is a questionnaire completed by care providers that can be very helpful in identifying motivating factors for an individual. The profile is derived from responses by the care providers and rank orders motivators for the person. The 15 motivations are Attention, Pain, Order, Morality, Physical Activity, Romance, Independence, Vengeance, Curiosity, Acceptance, Help Others, Frustration, Anxiety, Eating, and Social Contact. Obtaining these profiles can be extremely helpful in formulating hypotheses that can guide a behavior plan.

Plan Development. At this point it is important to address the hypothesized antecedents and the individual's "needs." A plan is developed to change the antecedents when possible and to help the person achieve the desired "needs" in a pro-social way. The emphasis is on ensuring positive and proactive approaches.

One intervention method is to identify an alternative behavior which can serve the same function as the target behavior in a pro-social way. A **replacement behavior** is a behavior that the individual can engage in to meet the same needs in a safe and socially appropriate manner. For example, if a person expresses a desire for self-harm when depressed (target behavior) in order to gain staff support and guidance (emotional need), he or she will be guided to ask the staff to talk and stay nearby for comfort (replacement behavior). It would not work to tell the person to use an independent coping strategy (relaxation, draw, etc.), if the need is to receive support and comfort from the staff. While socially appropriate and safe, it is not meeting the emotional need.

Plan Implementation. Before implementing any plan it is very important that everyone working with the person is in agreement with the steps of the plan. When multiple people are implementing a behavior plan it needs to be designed in a way that minimizes confusion. Consistency is essential for any plan. Just as the data collection system should be simple and easy, the behavior intervention plan needs to be simple and easy. In addition, everyone needs to be in agreement about the commitment to implementing the plan. It is not helpful to agree outwardly, but to do something different in practice. A mediocre plan implemented consistently is far better than a great plan implemented inconsistently. It only takes one person to deviate from the plan to confuse the individual and eliminate its effectiveness.

Data Collection. Data is collected when the plan has begun to be implemented. This is how change is monitored. Data is very important at this stage because sometimes change is marginal. Depending on the history of the behavioral challenge, minimal change may be highly significant. If a person's reaction to depression leads to hospitalization ten times in one year and six the next, this may not be noted as significant as the incidents are still occurring. However, this shows a 40% improvement.

Plan Effectiveness. The intervention plan is then monitored for effectiveness. "Effectiveness" is relative to the behavior and the setting. If a person reduces incidents of physical aggression by 50% in one month, this may be considered effective because it was a significant improvement in a short period of time. On the other hand, if a person reduces the number of suicide attempts by 50% (from six to three in a three month period), the plan may not be considered "effective" because the person's life was in danger three times. Many settings cannot maintain safety for that degree of dangerousness, and, therefore, the plan may be considered "ineffective."

If a behavior plan is not effective the support team assesses the plan for possible reasons. Some of those reasons may include:

- The plan was not implemented for a sufficient amount of time to assess effectiveness.
- The functional analysis was not comprehensive enough and factors were missed.
- There was inconsistent implementation of the plan by support staff.
- Too many variables were introduced at once (e.g., medication change, staff change, new approach to a behavior).
- There was lack of the individual's input into the development of the plan and the person's needs were not identified.

- There was a lack of positive reinforcement in the plan.
- Personal variables of those working with the person were not recognized (e.g., personality differences).
- There was insufficient emphasis on teaching replacement behaviors.
- The hypothesis of the function of the behavior was wrong.
- The plan was not realistic (too complicated, costly, or detailed).
- The plan included too much control by the staff, and the person had few choices.

Staff consistency is one of the most important factors in an effective plan. At the same time, each staff person is an individual with his or her own personality and interpersonal style. When developing a plan it is important for it to include steps that can be implemented consistently and allow for individual differences. Some common reasons a behavior plan is implemented inconsistently include staff individuality. However, this needs to be considered and respected. The following are some examples:

- The staff may not believe in the potential effectiveness of the plan.
- The staff may believe they have a more effective way of dealing with the behavior and do things differently when they are with that person.
- The plan may have been designed without enough input from the people who work most closely with the person.
- The staff may feel their input is not as important as the "specialist" who developed the plan.
- There may be cultural considerations among the staff that interfere with the implementation of the plan.
- The behavior may escalate before it gets better, and it may be difficult for the staff to tolerate an exacerbation of the behavior.
- The staff may be discouraged in dealing with a very challenging behavior with little improvement.
- There may not be enough people on the staff to implement the program effectively.
- The staff's feelings toward the individual may interfere with their ability to effectively implement the strategies.

- The staff may not agree philosophically with the intervention plan.
- There was not adequate training to allow the staff to implement the program effectively.
- Staff may not be able to see beyond the person's behavioral reputation to have any confidence that the behavioral strategies may work.
- The staff may believe rewards are a "bribe."
- The staff may fear if they have to do a "special plan" for one person, other people they work with will be jealous.
- The staff may be burned out from dealing with the behavior.

Encourage and listen to the support staff working with the individual. The support staff know the person better than most and have insights that are invaluable. Their insights are far past what behavior consultants or other "specialists" will gain in the short time they know the person. Often support staff defer to the specialists because they believe their knowledge is not as advanced and their insights are not valuable. That is simply not true. Without the knowledge and insights of the direct care staff a plan is not likely to be effective.

D-N-A

When designing a behavior plan, first, consider the **Developmental level (D)** of the individual. This includes the person's level of cognitive functioning as well as emotional functioning and maturity. It is important to know how the person processes information so the plan can be designed to emphasize the individual's strengths. For example, if the person has difficulty with communication the plan should emphasize visual modalities. It is also important to consider the person's developmental stage. For example, the person may desire increased independence or more peer relationships. It is also important to know what the individual's skill level is in taking on the new challenges so appropriate supports are provided.

Second, identify the **Need (N)** that is being met with the behavior. As discussed, if the person is not helped to find a safe and socially acceptable way to get that need met, the plan is less likely to work. The behavior generally serves a purpose and that purpose is important to the person. That needs to be respected.

Third, **Adapt (A)** the intervention to meet the developmental level. For example, if a person is feeling anxious and wanting attention from support staff, it may not be possible for the person to identify and use relaxation skills without support. Instead, establish a plan that supports the person in asking for or accepting help from a support person with guidance to identify a relaxing activity.

The Basics of Behavioral Theory

Thorndike (1911) was one of the early theorists interested in identifying the function and response of behavior. He stated in the "Law of Effect" that when an action is closely accompanied by a satisfying experience, the action and experience will be associated. He went on to define the "Law of Exercise" as when the connection between stimulus and response which become stronger through repetition. In other words, if an action is paired with something the person likes, the action will be associated with something positive. Further, if they are paired together frequently, the positive association will become stronger. The same can be said for traumatic experiences. The more frequently a person experiences an abusive response to a situation, the stronger the negative association will become. For example, if a person has experienced negative treatment by a caregiver, he or she will be more likely to have a negative reaction to future caregivers.

Skinner's (1953) theory was primarily focused on the way behavior affects the environment to produce consequences and the way favorable consequences, or reinforcement, work to increase the probability that a behavior will recur. Therefore, if a person uses screaming as a way to avoid taking a shower, screaming is more likely to continue if it is successful in helping to avoid the shower. The most common use of reinforcement is positive reinforcement. *Positive reinforcement* is a stimuli that increases the probability of a response when added to a situation. For example, a person is more likely to do chores for an allowance or call a friend who is funny. Positive reinforcement can work to increase a replacement behavior, but it can also work to reinforce a target behavior. For example, each time a woman takes a shower she gets to use special soaps that she likes. Theoretically, this is considered a favorable response and using the soap works to increase the number of showers. On the other hand, if she doesn't want to shower and gets out of doing so if she screams, the positive reinforcement of not showering increases the screaming. It is important to consider which outcome is desired and what is being reinforced.

There are two reinforcement schedules: continuous reinforcement and intermittent reinforcement. *Continuous reinforcement* involves a reinforcement schedule in which the reinforcement is delivered after every occurrence of the behavior; the reinforcer is continuous. Learning occurs more quickly when the reinforcer is continuous. *Intermittent reinforcement* involves a reinforcement schedule that is unpredictable; the reinforcer is intermittent. Learning occurs more slowly when a reinforcer is intermittent. Rewards provide a positive association to a taught behavior, which is why it is important to introduce a new skill with rewards. Once the behavior occurs more consistently and the person feels positively about it, the rewards can lessen.

While a behavior pattern is established more quickly with a continuous reinforcer, it is also the quickest to stop when the reinforcer is not there. A behavior pattern is established more slowly with intermittent reinforcement; however, it produces the most long-standing behavior change. It is very important to be aware of this because unwanted behavior patterns are most often reinforced intermittently. For example, if it is in the plan that a woman gets her favorite soaps when she showers, but not when she screams, it is only effective when all staff members working with her are consistent. If there is one staff person who either does not give her the soaps when she showered without screaming, or allows her to avoid the shower when she screams, it can establish a very strong behavior pattern because of the inconsistent reinforcement. Consistency among the people on the support team is very important. Remember, an "okay" plan implemented consistently is far better than a fabulous plan implemented inconsistently. Well-written behavior plans used inconsistently can become contaminated and unable to be used in the future.

A combination of both reinforcement schedules is most effective. When a change is introduced, continuous reinforcers are most effective. Then, as the behavior pattern is more established the number of times a reinforcer is provided is reduced. This transition is best when the value of the reinforcer increases as the frequency decreases. For example, if a man is able to go to the coffee shop of his choice with a favorite staff person after two days of attending day program, he can go to a professional baseball game with a favorite staff person after a month of attending day program. The change is not introduced until the behavior plan is well-established. It is very important the person feels successful and trusts that the positive outcome will occur.

Special Topics - A New View

There are some behavior patterns that tend to be viewed differently for individuals with an intellectual disability. This may be because their expressed needs are communicated with an unsafe or socially inappropriate behavior. The focus is then on the behavior, not the need. It also may be that because their skills and abilities are underestimated, challenges are not presented to them. A few of the common issues will be presented here with a new way of looking at them.

"Manipulative" Behavior. Often individuals with an intellectual disability find creative ways to get their needs met. If the way they choose is seen as frustrating by others it can be interpreted as "manipulative." Instead of emphasizing the annoyance of the behavior pattern, focus on the abilities an individual has in order to get needs met. It requires a lot of cognitive strengths and abilities for a person to be able to manipulate others. A person who is "manipulative" must also:

Be observant - to watch others to time the behavior correctly for the desired outcome

Be patient - to wait for the right person or time to engage in the behavior for the desired outcome

Possess foresight - to be able to plan into the future and foresee the outcome

Be socially skilled - to present the challenge in a way that it works (if it didn't work they wouldn't do it)

A person with these skills can set goals, make a plan, and have the patience to work toward the outcome. These are all important qualities in assisting someone in getting needs met.

"Attention-Seeking" Behavior. Individuals who are challenged with dual diagnoses typically need the support of others to help them cope. At the same time they may not have been taught the skills to communicate those needs in a way that works for the support team. Instead, they may choose crying, screaming, and provoking others as ways to bring attention to their needs. These choices are clearly bothersome to others and frustrating to the support person. It is common for the support person to say it is "just for attention." The support team may identify attention-seeking as the target behavior to be addressed. In fact, most people want attention at some time or other. Individuals with an intellectual disability typically choose methods that are common for their developmental level, not necessarily their chronological age. Their "attention-seeking" behaviors may, in fact, be appropriate for them. Before classifying a behavioral response of "attention-seeking" as inappropriate ask the following questions:

- Does the person have the skills to pro-socially communicate feelings and needs?
- Does the person have the ability to independently formulate options of coping skills when feeling overwhelmed?
- Is this person seeking interpersonal interactions because there are few opportunities for interactions otherwise?
- Has the person been alone for a long period of time?
- Is the person seeking external controls to manage the intense feelings of anxiety, depression, agitation, etc.?
- Does the person have the social skills to seek out appropriate social interactions?
- Are there activities that are cognitively and socially appropriate available to that individual?

If a person is needing attention from his or her support person for any of the mentioned reasons, simply telling the person to "wait" may only work for a brief time or not at all. On the other hand, if the reason he or she is seeking attention is addressed, the behavior challenge is less likely to occur. "Attention-seeking" behaviors can be described as anything from repetitive questions to aggression or self-injurious behaviors. If a person is feeling anxious and is managing ruminating thoughts by seeking interactions with repetitive questions, the behavior is likely to escalate if the focus is on the repetitive questions because the real reason for the behavior is not being addressed.

Individuals with dual diagnoses tend to need more attention and support to cope with the challenge of the mental health diagnosis. Due to the cognitive limitations that were described in Chapter 2, using coping skills independently is very challenging. To do so, they need to stay focused (attention), be able to identify which skills to use (long-term retrieval), and use self-talk to process and remember why using the skill is helpful (insight). This process requires executive functioning, which is a known weakness for individuals with an intellectual disability. Continuous staff support is often needed to compensate for these weaknesses. One strategy that can be effective when working with an individual who needs consistent and frequent staff support is to use "wow" papers. "Wow" papers are pieces of paper that are given to the individual with positive statements from the staff.

"Resistive" Behavior. The term "resistive" has been commonly used in behavior plans to represent anything from a person not doing what the staff ask to not accepting help when in an unsafe situation. This term should always be clarified. For example, at one point when a person was described as "resistive" it was synonymous with "non-compliant." Another time the behavior was considered "defiant." These terms are discouraged. While it sounds like the person is doing something wrong, it may only be a way for the person to communicate a choice.

Indeed, there are times when following staff instruction is very important. If a person has difficulty following staff or a care provider's instruction, it is recommended that the target behavior be termed more specifically. For example, if a person is walking out of the house unsupervised and does not return when asked, the target behavior may be bolting or wandering. If a person has decided not to take a shower for a week, a goal centered around a shower plan would be more appropriate.

Sexual Development. Disrobing in public, sexual promiscuity, and public masturbation are some examples of target behaviors that can be related to sexual development. Physical development as it relates to sexuality is chronologically the same for a person with an intellectual disability as it is for a typically developing adult. On the other hand, the understanding of sexuality is often very different.

Sexual development is often not discussed with individuals with an intellectual disability. When they are young it is often assumed they are too young and immature to understand. In addition, the focus is not on adulthood, but on providing the supports they need as children and adolescents. When they are adults, it is often assumed that someone has already discussed issues of sexuality. Therefore, the discussion and teaching are overlooked. Sometimes formal teaching about sexual development, puberty, body changes, privacy, and touch are never done.

The rate of sexual abuse among individuals with an intellectual disability is higher than the general population (Ryan, 1996). There are several hypothesized reasons. First, individuals with an intellectual disability often require help with personal care, such as showering and dressing. This leads to atypical experiences around privacy. Group home administrators will often comment on the short time the staff have to get to know the residents before they are helping them with self-care tasks. This sends the message that nudity and touch are not private. Second, individuals with an intellectual disability are encouraged to follow the instructions of the adults caring for them. If they are presented with a situation in which their bodies are not respected, such as with physical or sexual abuse, they may be less likely to know that it is wrong. This can make them very vulnerable. Third, adult relationships are often not developed typically. The opportunity for a healthy adult sexual relationship is more difficult to find and in some instances is discouraged. This limits the opportunity for experience and learning.

Given these circumstances, behaviors such as public nudity, disrobing, and masturbation are not interpreted the same way for someone with these atypical experiences. Education around sexual development and adult sexuality is very important for everyone, particularly those with target behaviors that include inappropriate sexual behaviors.

Leisure Skills. Leisure skills are important components in anyone's quality of life. Yet, they are very often overlooked for people with dual diagnoses. One reason is because their other challenges tend to overshadow leisure skills and place them as a lower priority. When someone is depressed and suicidal, one doesn't often think of helping them develop a hobby as a part of the treatment plan. When working with a depressed person in the general population, one of the things that is addressed is the loss of pleasure in activities the person previously found enjoyable. However, this is often not discussed with people who have an intellectual disability. In fact, often people with dual diagnoses do not engage in "leisure' activities. When asked to list what things they enjoy doing, this may include going to places they like, eating out, shopping, etc., but many times leisure activities or hobbies are not included.

Developing areas of interest is an important part of living a well-balanced life. For people with dual diagnoses, teaching them how to engage in leisure skills may be one of the main components of their treatment plan. Leisure skills can provide activities to help distract them from feeling depressed or anxious, add enjoyment to their life, increase independence, and provide structure during unstructured times.

Independently enjoying activities is a skill that needs to be developed for many people. It requires identifying an activity, organizing materials or time to engage in that activity, and learning new aspects as they advance in the activity. Considering the cognitive factors discussed, individuals may need some support in getting these activities started. They may need help purchasing supplies, identifying what they want to do, getting started, and scheduling time for the activity. It may take some time to get activities started, but in the long run these can provide tremendous sources of joy for people. Some ideas to get started:

- Making art (e.g., clay, painting, drawing)
- Jewelry making
- Collecting sports memorabilia
- Walking
- Listening to music
- Cooking
- Doing puzzles
- Dancing
- Learning math or a foreign language
- Studying maps
- Scrapbooking
- Making models
- Making greeting cards to send
- Doing arts and crafts

Chapter 7

Stress Among Individuals with an Intellectual Disability

Much has been written about the effects of stress on both physical and mental health. The research has discussed the factors which create stress and the factors which lessen it. However, the impact of stress on individuals with an intellectual disability is often overlooked and the findings from the stress management research have historically not been applied to this population. Yet, individuals with an intellectual disability face many potential sources of stress.

There are several concepts in the stress management research that are particularly relevant to this population. Before exploring those concepts, it is important to understand the stress experience. Stress as a concept is divided into two parts: the stressors and the response to stress. Sources of stress can be external, including environmental factors such as loud and chaotic environments, and experiences such as loss or trauma. It can also be a result of internal experiences such as cold, hunger, feeling ill, etc. The experience of stress is unique to each person. What is considered a stressor to one individual may not be a source of stress to another. Consequently, there is a considerable amount of individual variability in what is considered stressful and how stress is manifested.

Basic Stress Management Principles

The following are basic concepts from the stress management literature that have been applied to the general population. These concepts are often overlooked in their application for individuals with an intellectual disability.

Stress can occur in response to the level of stimulation in an environment.

Environments that are either too stimulating or not stimulating enough can be stressful. The experience of what is overstimulating or understimulating can vary among individuals. These two types of environments, at either end of the continuum, can impact an individual's mental and physical health. Either type of environment can produce distress.

The clustering of life events can increase susceptibility to illness. In 1967, Holmes and Rahe developed a rating scale called the Social Adjustment Rating Scale. It lists 43 different life events that include events such as the death of a spouse or family member, changing jobs, changes in living conditions, etc. Each event has a numerical value assigned to it which reflects the "average stressfulness" of each of the life events. Each event is rated from 0-100. The higher the rating scale, the higher the chance of illness and hospitalization within the year. Consequently, to introduce a lot of changes to a person's life at one time is not recommended, if it can be helped. Too many changes can increase the likelihood of illness or disease. Stress can reduce immune system functioning. It is interesting to note that even the word "disease" means "not at ease."

Stress can result from pleasant as well as unpleasant events. People often don't think about the fact that even good changes in someone's life can be stressful. Whether someone is excited because he is going to Disneyland or he is upset because he can't go to Disneyland, the body experiences a certain level of physical arousal. This arousal causes wear and tear on the body, although, there is some evidence that pleasant stress is not as harmful (Seyle, 1974). Additionally, some level of stress is needed to help motivate us to push ourselves.

Each person has limits of adaptability. The belief that someone should be able to adapt to a difficult environment if the desire and effort are present is simply not correct. Each person has his or her own limits.

Social support lessens stress. One of the variables which has been shown repeatedly throughout the stress management literature to buffer or lessen stress is social support.

Having too many choices can be stressful. Sometimes being presented with too many choices or options can be overwhelming and distressing. In 1980, Ferguson stated that the average person in the United States was exposed to 65,000 more stimuli in that year than someone who lived 100 years ago. Now considering that his statement was made almost 30 years ago, the amounts of stimuli we are exposed to have increased even more since then.

Each person has an individual stress profile. In the general population, stress can be manifested through behavioral, medical, or emotional expressions. Stress can be exhibited by showing changes in any of these categories or all of these categories. Each person's response to stress becomes as individualized as a finger print. Therefore, it is important to be aware of the warning signs that the person is becoming stressed so that either the source of stress can be addressed or coping skills can be used.

Implications

The principles discussed above all have implications for individuals with an intellectual disability. The following are suggested applications of some of these principles for working with this population::

Good fit. Finding a good fit between the level of stimulation in the environment and the person's needs is important. Since overstimulating or understimulating environments can cause stress, it is important to consider the match between the individual and the environment. Although overstimulating environments are often identified as triggering events for challenging behaviors among individuals with an intellectual disability, little attention is given to understimulating environments. Boredom can be stressful enough to trigger problem behaviors. Having little to do during the day can sometimes be an invitation for behavioral challenges to surface. The individual may seek to create activity or excitement in ways that are not adaptive or productive. For example, when exploring the reasons why a person may become aggressive, examine the activity level around the person at the time. Was the individual left alone with nothing to do? Were the people around the person so involved in the details of their daily lives that they weren't interacting with him or her? Sometimes a clue that the individual may be bored is the fact that the problem behaviors do not occur in environments where there is more activity. If this occurs, it is important to help ensure that the person has meaningful and interesting activities available. Observe the person's reactions and whether or not the type of activity or lack of activity triggers a problem behavior. Be mindful of any connection between the level of noise and activity in the environment and the person's reactions.

Transition slowly. Introduce changes gradually and try to avoid introducing too many changes at one time. Do not assume that if the person is cooperative with the changes that stress is not being experienced. All changes require adjustments, including mental, emotional, and physical adjustments. Individuals with an intellectual disability may need help spacing major changes in their lives so that they don't have to experience too many major life changes at one time. For example, if a person changes residences, this may also be accompanied by changes in the person's day program or vocational program. Often people with an intellectual disability move to different homes only to start new jobs or attend a new day programs within days of moving. For some, these changes may cause minimal stress. However, for others, it can be too stressful with too many changes that require both mental and physical adjustments. Most people in the general population would like to have the time to adjust and settle in to their new home before starting a new job. Yet this opportunity is not always given to those with an intellectual disability.

Be aware of physical illness. Pay attention to the signs and symptoms of physical illness. Since the stress produced by changes may increase susceptibility to illness, it is important to pay attention to changes in the individual's physical health. This becomes particularly important in working with people with an intellectual disability who are non-verbal. It is important for care providers or on-line staff to be vigilant to changes, even the slightest of changes, in the individual's behavior which may indicate a physical issue. If the person has changed residences, the people who may have cared for the person for years may no longer be involved in his or her life. Given the stress inherent in the move, coupled with new care providers who may not be aware of the person's usual indications of illness, it becomes even more important to be vigilant. When making this transition, it is helpful to get information from previous care providers regarding some of the typical symptoms the person may display when not feeling well.

Plan ahead. Help the person plan for events in ways that reduce stress. As behavioral consultants, we have frequently encountered situations in which an individual with an intellectual disability becomes very excited about an upcoming social event or outing. Often, staff or care providers feel as though they can't tell the individual about the event too far in advance. Otherwise the person becomes very agitated, even though the outing being scheduled is positive. Pleasant events can be stressful because they also can result in an increase arousal to the nervous system. Therefore, it is important to consider the impact that even pleasant events can have and to introduce those events in ways that minimize the person's stress level.

Comfort zones. Learn about the person's comfort zones. The belief that someone should be able to adapt to a difficult environment if he or she just tries hard enough is not correct. Each person has his or her own limits. Consequently, when someone with an intellectual disability is not responding well to certain stressors, there may be a tendency by others to want to reward the person for trying harder and for displaying the "appropriate" behaviors. Perhaps, the strategy should be to examine the pressures that the individual is facing and assist in removing these stressors rather than continuing to push the limits.

Social support. Help individuals maintain their social support networks and establish new social outlets. Individuals with an intellectual disability often do not have outlets to develop friendships. If they do develop some friendships, it is not unusual to lose them if they change residences. Since social support can help buffer or lessen stress, it is important to help them maintain or build their social support networks. Facilitating contact with family members and finding social activities to attend, such as dances, clubhouses, and sporting events, can decrease a sense of isolation. It is important to also focus on the quality of those social contacts and help individuals establish healthy social boundaries. However, social contacts also have the ability to create stress if the social contacts and relationships create problems.

Routines. Help individuals to establish routines. Daily routines add a rhythm and predictability to our lives. This can help to lessen anxiety, facilitate a sense of control, and help us to meet daily demands. Helping individuals with an intellectual disability establish a routine removes some of the need for executive functioning which is a known cognitive weakness among this population. Reducing that extra pressure can be calming.

Avoid too many choices. We may have the best of intentions in trying to ensure that individuals with an intellectual disability have the opportunities that we are afforded. However, in doing so, it is important to consider how to do this. Opportunities should be presented in ways that are measured and thoughtful and do not overwhelm them with choices.

Importance of Considering Stress Management Principles

One of the reasons this chapter is so important is because people with dual diagnoses are often faced with situations that would cause stress for most people. The difference is that most adults can either change some aspect of the situation or use cognitive coping skills to deal with it if they can't evoke any situational changes. How we view a situation can influence our stress level. In other words, if we are not able to change a situation, we are left to change our cognitive appraisal of the situation. For example, if we are in traffic we can start thinking about how terrible it is that we can't get home on time or how the traffic is a huge inconvenience. This type of thinking will lead to more stress. If we can't change the situation, i.e., we can't control the traffic, we can modify our thoughts about it and which can lessen our stress. Since individuals with an intellectual disability may not have the ability to change their cognitive appraisals, they are even more likely to experience increased stress.

Not only is cognitive appraisal an important element in stress management, but the issue of control over one's environment is also an important mediator of stress. Even though people are faced with stressful situations, if they feel they have control over aspects of their environment it can lessen the stress response. Since many individuals with an intellectual disability have little, or perhaps no control, over their environmental circumstances, their level of stress can remain high and prolonged. This can have an adverse impact on their physical health as well as their mental health. Therefore, appreciating the concepts derived from the stress management literature and research and their applicability to the lives of individuals with an intellectual disability cannot be overstated.

Chapter 8

Transitional Planning

Individuals with an intellectual disability may find themselves facing numerous changes in their lives with regard to their living arrangements. If the person is moving from one setting to another, the success in adjusting to the move can be strongly influenced by the quality of the transitional or discharge plan. If the move occurs quickly without proper preparation, it can be a formula for a behavioral and/or psychiatric crisis or a placement failure. It can also become a crisis for the care providers or individuals who support the person. The following sections provide recommendations for transitional planning based on a variety of potential living arrangements. Since each state differs in the options available for individuals with an intellectual disability, the following information is presented in an effort to cover transitions from a variety of living arrangements and along a continuum of care.

Transitional Planning from an Institutionalized Setting to a Community Residence

Transitional planning (i.e., discharge planning) really begins when the individual is admitted to a facility. Criteria for discharge should be identified upon admission. For discharge to be considered, the behaviors which led to the individual's admission should no longer be occurring with a level of intensity or frequency that the person could not live safely in the community. This includes the family home, group home, supported living apartment, or in any other living arrangement in the community.

Since the individual is being discharged from a highly structured setting, it is particularly important to ensure that the proper supports and services have been identified to facilitate a move back to the community. It is important to use a multi-disciplinary treatment team approach. This type of approach involves obtaining input from professionals from different disciplines, such as medical, social work, psychology, nutrition, and speech therapy, as well as direct care staff and family members. This ensures that important areas of the individual's life have received the appropriate attention and that the discharge plans are comprehensive. Obtaining information in the following areas can ensure that the right supports and services are available to assist the person in the transition. All of the questions in this section are included in the Transitional Planning and Preparation Form provided in Appendix D of this book. The form is provided as the framework to gather information when planning a transition from an institutionalized setting to a community residence. However, this form can be used as the framework when planning a transition from any living setting to another living setting.

Placement history. It is important to review an individual's past living arrangements and whether or not those types of arrangements were successful. This type of review can provide information regarding the types of living arrangements that did not work for the person, so that mistakes are not repeated. For example, if an individual lived in group homes or adult residential facilities and received discharge notices from all of the homes due to challenging behaviors, then it is important to look at why those living arrangements were unsuccessful. Was it because there were too many people living in the home and the individual did not like living with that many people? Did this serve as a trigger for some of the behavioral challenges? Was it the mix of personalities in the home? Was it because there was not enough supervision or structure in the home? Did the person's mental health needs exceed the capability of the care providers to provide the necessary care? Does the person need to avoid congregate living arrangements and live in an apartment with supervision?

With this type of review, new living arrangements can be identified that can help the person to be more successful. After all, Albert Einstein once said that the definition of insanity is doing the same thing over and over again and expecting different results.

The following questions can be helpful in providing this type of review:

1. What were the individual's previous living arrangements? This should include the type of living arrangements and the length of time the individual resided in each place.
2. Were any of the living arrangements successful for the individual? Which arrangements were best and why did the person have to leave?
3. Which living arrangements were unsuccessful? What happened and why didn't they work?
4. If the individual has the verbal skills, can he or she identify a preferred living situation? If this arrangement is not feasible due to the person's medical and/or behavioral challenges, what would it take to help the person reach the goal?
5. If the person is currently residing in an institution, how long has it been since the individual lived in the community? If the individual is not ready to move to the community, what skills or types of supports are needed in order to support a discharge from the institution?
6. If living in an institutionalized setting, has the person ever had to change units or residences within the facility? Was the change the result of the individual's behaviors or medical needs and how did the person adjust to the change? Did the change result in an increase in behavioral challenges or an increase in psychiatric symptoms?
7. Does the individual's family support a move to the community and to a less structured setting? If not what are the family's concerns?
8. Does the individual have a history of psychiatric hospitalizations? If so, how frequent were the hospitalizations and what prompted the admissions?

Developmental history. Obtaining a developmental history can be important in discovering the cause of the intellectual disability. Was it the result of a head injury? Was it the result of a genetic disorder or did the individual suffer a stroke as a child? Is there even an identified cause? This information is very important in determining if some of the behavioral challenges or psychiatric symptoms can be linked to the events which caused the intellectual disability. This can have important implications for treatment strategies and behavioral interventions. For example, an individual with fetal alcohol syndrome may be more likely to be impulsive or easily agitated. Additionally, if the individual has a syndrome that caused the intellectual disability, it is important to know if the syndrome is likely to cause deteriorations in the individual's health status or cognitive functioning abilities. This has implications for the types of supports the individual may need in future living arrangements.

The following are some of the questions to be considered in reviewing a person's developmental history:

1. What is the cause of the individual's intellectual disability? Is a syndrome involved? If so, does that syndrome have behavioral or medical symptoms that need to be considered in placement planning?
2. Does the person have a diagnosis in the autistic spectrum that has implications for the type of living arrangements and environmental surroundings?

Communication abilities. Behavioral challenges are more likely to occur among individuals who lack a formal communication system. Therefore, it is important to understand how an individual currently communicates his or her desires, wants, needs, etc. It is important to facilitate the person's ability to communicate to others and facilitate the ability of others to understand the individual. When meeting new people we rely on asking and answering questions to get to know them. We are less likely to ask questions when we feel insecure. So when an individual moves from a very structured, familiar setting of an institution to a lesser structured, unfamiliar group home, being able to communicate with that person, either verbally or non-verbally, is essential in creating a more soothing environment for the person. For example, if the person relies on American Sign Language (ASL) or a picture communication system, then it is important that future living arrangements include staff training in that particular communication system.

The following are some aspects of communication that should be considered in the transitional planning:

1. What is the extent of the individual's expressive language? How does the person currently communicate wants, needs, preferences, dislikes, etc? Is it through purposeful reach, pointing, or verbally?
2. Does the individual use any communication device or any communication system that would require training for future care providers?

3. Does the person have any hearing deficits that impact communicative abilities?

4. Does the person use ASL or unique manual signs?

5. What is the individual's receptive language skill level? Can the person understand basic verbal instructions and do instructions and questions need to be presented in a certain way? For example, should communications be provided by care providers using concrete, short sentences with no more than one-step instructions provided at any given time?

6. Does the individual exhibit episodes of prolonged or loud vocalizations that could be disruptive to others in the home or the neighbors?

7. How does the individual communicate when in pain?

Social. Social factors become important to consider in identifying appropriate future living arrangements for a person. For example, does the person enjoy living with several other people, or is a congregate living situation likely to result in an increase in mental health issues or behavioral challenges? If the person is going to be living with other people who have dual diagnosis, it is important to consider the mix of personalities in the home. For example, if the individual is a private person who doesn't like people to intrude upon his or her physical space, having the person live with someone who is physically intrusive may be problematic. If the individual is very social and active, he or she may not want to be around people who tend to be quiet, withdrawn, or not interested in participating in activities in the community. Examining the social needs of the person can help to identify the type of living arrangement that is most suitable.

It is important to also identify the relationships that are important to the individual so that efforts can be made to help the person maintain those relationships. There have been many situations in which the person has sabotaged a new living arrangement because of missing previous care providers or family members. It is important to identify the individual's support system and important social contacts.

The following are questions to ask in assessing the social needs and the types of social supports needed as an individual changes residential settings:

1. Does the person enjoy being alone? How social is the person?

2. Does the individual enjoy spending time with care providers and/or peers?

3. Who is included in and extent of the person's current support system?
4. What kind of peer group does the individual need?
5. Does the person respond better to male or female care providers?
6. Does the person want to leave his or her current social support system?
7. Is the family in contact with the individual? If so, to what degree are they in contact and are those relationships conflictual?
8. To what extent does the person need assistance from care providers to facilitate social relationships?

Individual likes and dislikes. One of the difficulties commonly encountered among individuals with an intellectual disability is their lack of leisure skills and hobbies. This can create boredom and a lack of structure that may lead to behavioral challenges and an increase in some psychiatric issues. For example, out of boredom an individual may engage in some negative behaviors to get attention from care providers. A person who suffers from anxiety may have more of an opportunity to worry when there is nothing else to do to occupy his or her time. Consequently, it is important for those people who support individuals with an intellectual disability to help them participate in the things they enjoy, promote greater access to new experiences so they can expand their interests, and help increase their independence in these areas. When considering placements, it is important to match the level of desired activity of the person with what is offered at the home. When care providers complain about the "neediness" of the residents they support, it is often because there is a mismatch in what the residents are seeking and the activities that are provided. Consider the following areas with regard to interests and leisure activities:

1. What are the individual's likes and dislikes?
2. What kind of community activities does the person enjoy?
3. Currently, what is the frequency with which the person accesses activities in the community?
4. Does the person exhibit any behavioral challenges while in the community that may require enhanced supervision?
5. What kind of leisure skills and hobbies does the person have? What does the person enjoying doing with his or her free time?

6. Does the individual need the support of care providers to engage in these hobbies or leisure activities?
7. Does the person need a very active daily schedule or does the person prefer to be more sedentary?

Self-help skills. Identifying the individual's level of independence with regard to the activities of daily living is important in identifying the appropriate living arrangements. Activities of daily living include toileting, dressing, grooming, bathing, and eating. Identifying the types of supports the individual needs in these areas is important for determining staffing patterns and demands on potential care providers. For example, if an individual needs a significant amount of help eating, dressing, and bathing, this needs to be considered in identifying the type of residential resource that can provide that level of care. The following are some of the questions to consider in identifying community resources that can provide the appropriate care for the individual:

Toileting
1. With regard to toileting, is the individual continent? What level of assistance does the person need with toileting needs?
2. Does the person have issues with constipation that require such interventions as the administration of a suppository? If so, would this require a certain level of nursing care in the residence?
3. Is there a history of nighttime incontinence that would require a care provider to assist the individual during the night?
4. Does the person exhibit any behavioral challenges around toileting that would require enhanced care provider supervision, such as smearing feces, compulsively flushing the toilet, or flooding the bathroom by turning on the faucets, etc.?

Grooming/bathing/dressing
1. With regard to grooming, bathing, and dressing, what level of assistance does the person require from care providers (e.g., verbal prompts, hand-over-hand assistance, total care, etc.)?
2. How cooperative is the individual in performing self-care tasks? If care provider assistance is needed, does the person refuse assistance or become combative? Is self-care assistance going to be potentially time consuming for a care provider?
3. Does the person have a seizure disorder which would require monitoring while showering to ensure safety?

4. Does the individual need adaptive equipment for any of the self-care tasks such as a pedestal bath, etc.?

5. Does the person display any tactile defensiveness which increases resistiveness when care providers try to assist?

6. What is the individual's current schedule or routine with regard to these activities? For example, does the person prefer to take a shower in the morning or evening? Is it important to maintain the current routine?

7. Are there any clothing preferences? For example, does the person dislike wearing shoes with laces?

8. Are there any compulsive or ritualistic behaviors exhibited by the individual around any of the self-care tasks that interfere with the completion of the tasks?

Eating

1. What level of assistance is required around eating? Is the individual independent with eating?

2. Does the person have any unsafe eating habits such as eating too quickly, eating too much, or stealing food? Would any of these unsafe eating habits pose a health and safety risk to the individual if not carefully monitored? Does the person require enhanced supervision during mealtimes? Does the individual have any choking risks due to unsafe eating habits or due to dysphagia that would required either special diets and/or special monitoring? Do any facility modifications need to be made to the residence or facility prior to the individual moving in?

3. Have there been any issues around food that have been problematic for the individual, such as compulsively drinking water (i.e., psychogenic polydypsia) or an eating disorder?

Medical considerations. An individual's medical conditions and medical needs are very important to consider in determining the level of care and the type of community residence that is needed. For example, does the individual need nursing services for insulin injections? Identifying the current medical conditions, including any sensory deficits, becomes critical to ensuring that the appropriate level of care is provided. Considering sensory deficits, such as vision problems, helps to ensure that appropriate environmental modifications are also made, if needed. It is important to consider any vision problems and difficulties with ambulation in order to create an environment that is safe for the individual. If the person is prone to falls due to orthopedic or neurological issues, then it is important to ensure that the environment is safe. Large, bulky furniture items should be out of the way so that the individual does not trip. Flooring should not be so smooth or slippery that it increases the risk of slipping or falling. Carpets may be helpful in providing more traction for the individual, whereas, throw rugs may increase the risk of tripping. Special consideration may need to be given with regard to how the individual's bedroom is arranged. For example, if the person gets up at night and gets out of bed without assistance, is there a likelihood of bumping into the dresser if it is too close to the bed? For an individual who is prone to falls and fractures, because of medical conditions such as osteoporosis, a fall could result in broken bones.

It is also important to consider the individual's dietary and nutritional needs. For example, does the individual need to be fed via a feeding tube? Does the diet need to be modified to a chopped or pureed diet? This has implications for not only the type of facility that is identified, since not all residences may be able to do tube feedings, but it also has implications for staff training. For example, if the person is to receive a ground diet, it is important that staff be trained in how to prepare the meals to ensure the proper consistency. It is also important that any food allergies be identified.

The following are areas to consider to ensure that the proper supports and services are provided based on an individual's medical needs:

Current medical conditions
1. What are the individual's current medical conditions and does the person require specialized care such as nursing services?
2. Are the conditions currently symptomatic or asymptomatic and what level of monitoring is required?
3. Are there any medical conditions which are progressive? Is the person's health status likely to deteriorate in the near future? If so, would the individual's health care needs exceed the living arrangement currently being considered?
4. Have there been any recent hospitalizations? If so, is the person medically stable enough to consider a move?
5. When the individual has been ill, is there a history of quickly succumbing to the illness with a slow recovery?
6. Does the person have any current medical conditions that may be exacerbated by the stress of a move? For example, does the individual have high blood pressure or any cardiac issues

that may be impacted by stress? Does this require special monitoring or follow-up?

7. Are there any medical conditions that are considered restricted health care conditions in the community and require specific health care plans that need to be reviewed by a local licensing agency?

8. Does the individual have any conditions that can be contagious to others, such as a form of hepatitis? Are there additional vaccinations required for the people working with the individual?

9. If the individual moves to the community, how readily available are the community medical resources and supports? Is gaining access to these supports going to be difficult?

10. Are there any past medical conditions that may re-occur? If so, what were the signs and symptoms exhibited by the individual when ill? What treatments were provided and were they effective?

11. Does the individual have a seizure disorder? How well controlled are the seizures and what types of interventions have been needed? For example, does oxygen need to be available or has the individual required injections in response to multiple seizures or status epilepticus?

12. With regard to motor skills, is the person able to walk independently? Is assistance required from others and what degree of assistance is needed?

13. Does the individual have an unsteady gait which increases the likelihood of falls?

14. Does the individual have any visual impairments, and if so, what is the extent of the vision difficulties? Does this require any environmental modifications?

15. Are there any sensory integration issues that require environmental modifications?

16. Are there any special dietary or nutritional supports required?

Behavioral challenges. Identifying the behavioral challenges presented by an individual is one of the most important variables to consider in identifying an appropriate community living arrangement. This is the second most important category to consider next to an individual's medical needs. If the person presents with significant behavioral challenges that exceed the resources of a community residence, or the ability of a family to provide needed supports, the living arrangement may be in jeopardy. This could lead to consequences such as behavioral crises, failed residential placements and injuries to the person or to care providers. Consequently, it is very important to consider a host of factors when identifying the services needed to support someone with dual diagnoses. The extent of the behavioral challenges and mental health needs will help determine staffing ratios, level of supervision, and level of training needed for care providers. The following are areas to consider in order to determine the proper supports and services needed to address the behavioral challenges:

1. What are the individual's current behavioral challenges? How frequently do they occur and how severe are they?
2. Are there identifiable antecedents or precursors?
3. Are there any restrictive interventions or devices being used to address the behaviors that would not be allowed in a community facility due to licensing regulations? This would include various forms of restraints such as wrist-to-waist restraints, helmets, etc. Can the use of these devices be faded out or discontinued prior to the individual leaving an institutionalized setting?
4. What are the histories of these behaviors? How long have they been occurring?
5. Are there any "behavioral alerts" (i.e., challenging behaviors that have not been identified as specific target behaviors, since they do not occur with sufficient intensity or severity to warrant and intervention)? These would include any behaviors that staff working in an institution encounter on a day-to-day basis, or encounter so frequently that they take them for granted. However, these behaviors if exhibited in a less structured or less restrictive setting, such as the community, may pose a problem.
6. Do any of the behavioral challenges impact participation in community outings or attendance at a day program?
7. Since old behavioral challenges can resurface under stress, what is the history of the behavioral challenges?
8. How does the person respond to change? Does it increase the frequencies or severities of the behavioral challenges?
9. What interventions, both proactive and reactive strategies, have been used to address the behavioral challenges?

10. Does the person have a psychiatric diagnosis? How are the symptoms of the psychiatric condition being addressed? Is the psychiatric condition being considered in creating the treatment goals or in creating any of the behavioral intervention plans?
11. Does the person currently suffer from insomnia or have a history of insomnia that may reoccur with the stress of a move? What level of staffing or supervision does this require?
12. If the person is aggressive, how frequent are the episodes of aggression and how intense are the incidents? Have they resulted in any injuries to the person or to others? What level of staffing is needed to intervene and de-escalate the behaviors?
13. Does the individual have a trauma history and if so, in what type of environment did the trauma occur? What type of trauma was it (e.g., sexual abuse, physical abuse)?

If an individual has been living in an institutionalized setting, and the frequencies of his/her behavioral challenges are low, it is important to consider whether or not the improvements are the result of environmental controls or the acquisition of new skills. Has the person actually learned more effective ways of getting needs met, coping with situations, etc., or have the behaviors improved because the people working with the individual have learned to avoid the triggers for the behaviors? This is critical to identifying the supports and services that will be needed in the community. If the problematic behaviors have stopped or decreased because the current environment has been able to introduce certain controls, it may be important to create similar types of environmental controls in the new residence.

Transitional planning team meetings. Based on the information obtained from the various categories during the assessment process, potential living arrangements can be identified for the individual. Once a potential care provider or living arrangement has been identified, transitional planning becomes very important in supporting the individual's move from an institutionalized setting to the community. In preparation for the individual's discharge from the facility, it is important to provide a forum for the care provider(s) to receive information about the individual's health status and conditions, behavioral issues, and the information obtained from the various assessment categories (i.e., self-help skills, likes/dislikes, social and leisure activities, communication skills, etc.). This can be accomplished by meeting with the individual's interdisciplinary treatment team. Currently, in the state of California, such meetings are referred to by various names, such as Transitional Supports Planning Team Meeting (TSM) or Initial Planning Team Conferences. Whatever the meeting is titled, it is important to meet and identify the appropriate supports and services needed to ensure that the individual's needs will be met once he or she moves. The meeting also becomes a forum for discussing the logistics of the move to the community, such as time frames, and the number of visits to the home to be arranged prior to the move, etc. By the end of the meeting, it is important to establish the following:

1. *Identify the type of living arrangement along with the level of staffing and supervision that is needed, based on the individual's behavioral challenges and medical needs.*

2. *Given the individual's medical conditions, identify the types of medical follow-up and consultations that are needed.* For example, if the individual has seizures, periodic consultations with a neurologist should be scheduled. As part of the discussion of medical needs, it is also important to discuss whether or not an individual is cooperative with medical appointments and procedures. Resistiveness or avoidance due to anxiety can adversely impact the quality of medical care and medical follow-up in the community. Some individuals have histories of refusing to attend medical appointments or they have needed sedation for the appointments. Some have needed restraint devices for medical procedures, such as soft tie restraints, or have had to undergo general anesthesia for examinations. Consequently, sedation may be needed for future medical appointments.

All current medical conditions should be identified. Obtain information on any previous medical conditions that may re-emerge and the signs and symptoms the individual exhibited when he or she had the condition. This becomes particularly important when working with individuals who do not possess expressive language skills. In addition, it is important to identify whether or not the individual has any current medical conditions that are likely to progress and how they may be managed.

3. *Identify any behavioral challenges and discuss the types of behavioral and psychological supports that will be needed.* This should include an identification of all of the challenging behaviors, and the environments and interpersonal situations that can trigger the behaviors. Also

discuss the strategies used by the staff to intervene, including the strategies that have been effective as well as the strategies to be avoided. Reviewing past problematic behaviors that have not been exhibited in awhile can be beneficial since these behaviors may re-surface during the stress of a move (i.e., known as stress induced regressions). When an individual is experiencing stress and the current stressors exceed their coping skills, past behaviors can re-emerge that were once part of the individual's behavioral repertoire. A behavioral history can be helpful in providing some of this information.

Information regarding any psychiatric diagnoses that have been identified should also be discussed. Is the individual currently experiencing any psychiatric symptoms and have there been any recent psychotropic medication changes? If the individual is receiving psychotropic medications for either the treatment of a psychiatric condition, or to address behavioral challenges, it is recommended that a move not occur in the midst of medication changes. Medication titrations (i.e., changes in dosage whether increases or decreases) have the potential for de-stabilizing behaviors. Therefore, introducing significant changes in the individual's life at the same time that medication changes are being introduced can complicate the situation. It can also cause confusion as to whether any regression is because of the medication change or whether it was the stress of the move.

4. *Review information about the individual's likes, dislikes, strengths, and needs.* This is important in ensuring that the individual is provided with access to enjoyable activities and life enriching activities. Reviewing this information can also provide care providers with opportunities to learn more about the individual and his or her strengths. Too often information focuses on the individual's behavioral challenges without a focus on strengths, attributes, and interests.

5. *Identify self-care strengths and needs.* This helps to identify the level of assistance the individual will need in performing activities of daily living. It is also an opportunity to identify any adaptive equipment that the individual may need, such as a shower chair or a divided dish for mealtimes in order to prevent spillage. Of particular importance is the need to review any unsafe eating habits, since these can increase the risk of choking. This also helps to identify the level of supervision needed around mealtimes.

6. *Identify the individual's methods of communication and communication skills.* At the end of the meeting, potential care providers should know how the individual communicates. Of particular importance, how the person indicates when in pain or discomfort?

7. *Identify leisure skills.* Information obtained in this area will help the care provider offer the types of opportunities the individual enjoys and also help to encourage the development of hobbies and more interests. This is important because unstructured time or "down time" can be an invitation for challenging behaviors to emerge.

8. *Review the day program and vocational needs.* It is important to discuss the individual's day program or vocational needs and ensure an appropriate fit between the individual's interests, skills, needs, and community resources. Since individuals who are moving from an institution to a community setting are used to a high amount of structure, having unstructured days can be a difficult transition. Therefore, it is important to assess the person's vocational needs and ensure that the opportunities to participate in a day program or vocational program are available, as soon as the person is ready to attend. Participation also provides increased social outlets and opportunities.

9. *Assess for social and cultural influences, values, and traditions.* This should include cultural traditions, such as food, routines, holidays, and activities. It should also include the person's religious beliefs and whether or not the individual wants to attend religious services.

Transitional Planning from One Adult Residential Facility to Another Adult Residential Facility

If another residential living arrangement is being sought as a result of the individual's behavioral challenges, it sometimes occurs in response to a placement crisis. The person may have received a discharge notice from one residence or facility due to behavioral challenges and a new residence needs to be located quickly. This type of move may occur with minimal, if any, transitional planning. Without proper preparation, future behavioral and/or psychiatric crises may occur again. This can lead to a long and varied placement history for the individual. In order to decrease the likelihood of another unsuccessful move, it is helpful to consider the following:

- What behaviors or situations led to the discharge notice?
- What intervention strategies were used to address the challenging behaviors in the previous residence, or other residences, and why were they ineffective? What can be done differently in the new home?

- Do the behaviors signal a possible underlying psychiatric disorder which has not yet been treated? Is this why the behaviors did not respond to behavioral interventions or other interventions?
- Was the placement unsuccessful because of staffing issues, i.e., staff responses or personalities, or staffing ratios?
- Did the individual want to continue living at the previous residence? If not, why did the person want to leave? Was the individual exhibiting challenging behaviors as a way to secure a change of residence?
- Were there conflicts among the residents at the home?
- If the current move is occurring because of increased behavioral challenges, have the factors which contributed to or caused the behavioral problems been identified? What types of stressors may have led to the behavioral regression? If so, what can be done to help reduce the individual's stress level?

If the move is to happen quickly, and there is little time to gather and pass on this type of information, then at a minimum, it is important that new care providers or staff receive at least the following information:

- The individual's likes and dislikes
- The person's psychiatric diagnosis and what that means for the individuals supporting the person
- A list of the challenging behaviors, the situations that trigger them, how to avoid those triggers, and how to react to the behaviors when they occur
- Information regarding any medical conditions or issues
- Self-help skills, including a list of what the individual can do without assistance or what level of assistance is needed
- Medications
- Day program information
- Current social support network, including family contacts and family involvement
- How the person communicates his or her needs

All of this information is important for care providers so they can try to avoid potential triggers for any challenging behaviors and more effectively meet the person's needs.

Transitional Planning from a Family Home to an Adult Residential Facility

The first out-of-home placement can be very difficult for a family. There are many feelings which can accompany this decision including guilt, frustration, and anxiety. The decision to find a residential program or facility usually occurs when the individual's needs exceed what a family can provide. Although these situations can be very difficult, they can also be beneficial for all concerned. Sometimes it is difficult for a family to provide the right amount of structure, environmental stimulation, and supervision. With enhanced intervention and supervision, the individual's behaviors or medical conditions may improve. When an out-of-home placement is sought, one of the most helpful strategies to adopt is that of teamwork. When families and the administrator and staff from a program work together it can greatly benefit the individual. One of the most difficult situations occurs when the family and the staff are in conflict and their interactions become negative and adversarial. Communication is the key. Although the staff at the residence provide different support than the love that the family can provide, this can be advantageous in that their observations may be more objective. Since they do not have the same long-standing emotional investment of families, they may be able to more clearly see the dynamics that could be contributing to some of the behavioral challenges. At the same time, families also have a history and an extensive knowledge of the person. Both parties bring significant information and important perspectives to the situation. Therefore, the following suggestions are provided to help foster a positive working relationship between families and care providers:

1. Visits with the family should be structured in ways that are the most helpful for the individual with the intellectual disability. For example, if the individual has a difficult time going back to the family home for a visit, perhaps the visit should occur at the individual's new home or in the community.
2. If a family member has concerns about the treatment of the person, this should be discussed with the home's administrator or other care providers. Identify whether or not it is simply a difference in approach and explore the rationale for the approach. If it is clearly maltreatment, it not only needs to be addressed but it may also need to be reported to the appropriate agencies.

3. It can sometimes be helpful if parents or involved family members attend medical appointments with the individual. They can provide history and information that the care providers may not have. The individual may also be more comfortable attending doctor appointments with family members and this could help to ease anxiety and decrease any resistiveness.

Transitional Planning from an Inpatient Psychiatric Setting to an Adult Residential Facility

The transitional planning and the comprehensiveness of the planning will vary depending upon the length of stay in the psychiatric hospital and the purpose of the hospitalization. Length of hospital stays can vary depending upon the reason for admission. Sovner, Beasley, and Desnoyers-Hurley (1995) proposed a subtyping of psychiatric admissions according to the following categories:

Type I Hospitalization

The duration of the stay for this type of hospitalization is usually anywhere from 3-14 days. This type of hospitalization is usually for individuals who have psychiatric diagnoses that are already established and they may be experiencing some acute symptoms or medication side effects. This type of admission is usually meant to be a short-term stay with the purpose of introducing medication changes or introducing a specific type of treatment.

Type II Hospitalization

During this type of hospital stay, the admission has been sought because of dangerous or out-of-control behaviors. The individual may have been at risk for harm to self or others. The length of the hospitalization may extend from 1-3 weeks with the goal of stabilizing the behaviors and formulating at least a provisional psychiatric diagnosis, if the behaviors are believed to be the result of an underlying psychiatric condition.

Type III Hospitalization and Type IV Hospitalization

This type of hospital stay can extend from 4-6 weeks. This can occur when a psychiatric diagnosis has not yet been determined. The admission will help to identify whether or not the behaviors are reflective of an underlying psychiatric condition. If so, treatment can be initiated, including monitoring of whether or not the medication trial is effective. This type of admission requires detailed monitoring of behaviors.

Discharge planning (i.e., transitional planning for psychiatric hospital discharges). Depending upon the length of stay, there may be little time for discharge planning or transition planning, particularly if another living arrangement needs to be identified just prior to discharge. A short term hospitalization may have been needed to address the immediate dangers of aggressive or self-injurious behavior. This often results in some psychotropic medication changes, or simply containment, followed by a discharge back to the community residence after a few days. In this type of situation, time is of the essence and the following is recommended:

1. Individuals in the person's support network, such as an interdisciplinary treatment team, should convene as soon as possible to review the events which precipitated the hospitalization. Was it a behavioral incident and what triggered the behavioral crisis? If the individual lives in a group home, board and care, or an adult residential facility, and a behavior plan was written, the plan should be reviewed to determine if any modifications need to be made and any intervention strategies provided to the staff.

2. Assess for any stressors in the individual's life that led to the hospitalization. Assist the individual in problem-solving strategies if there was a problem that contributed or caused the admission.

3. Schedule a follow-up meeting with the outpatient treating psychiatrist within a few days of the individual's discharge from the hospital. The coordination of care with other service providers, such as an outpatient treating psychiatrist, is very important. If possible, it is always helpful to try and facilitate the coordination of care between the inpatient psychiatrist and outpatient psychiatrist before discharge.

4. Immediately follow-up with any medical appointments if a medical condition was identified at the hospital or if an existing condition has been exacerbated.

5. If the individual has received a discharge notice from the residence while in the psychiatric hospital, this often creates an emergency placement situation for a service coordinator (i.e., social worker) if an agency is involved in supporting the individual. If a new residence can be located that will accept the person, he or she may move directly into that home upon discharge. As with any emergency discharge notice, the more

information that can be provided to the new care provider, the more proactive and effective they can be in providing the appropriate supports and avoiding any psychiatric, behavioral, or medical crises.

Whether the person is leaving a state institution, a psychiatric facility, or moving from one residence to another, knowledge and preparation are key. The more information that can be shared with potential care providers, the greater the likelihood that the appropriate supports and services will be in place. Too often, individuals with dual diagnoses have tumultuous placement histories that can contribute to feelings of anxiety, a lack of stability, and a decreased sense of control. Greater thoughtfulness and preparation with regard to their needs and their living arrangements can only help to increase their sense of safety, security, and success.

Chapter 9

Therapy for Individuals with Dual Diagnoses

Therapy is one of the main interventions and supports for individuals coping with psychiatric disorders. At the same time, traditional therapy often needs to be adapted when working with a person with an intellectual disability. It is incorrect to assume that because individuals have an intellectual disability they are not able to successfully participate in therapy. Many of the traditional interventions can be very effective for this group of people. At the same time, the presentation of the information will be more effective if it is adapted to account for the cognitive ability, communication skills, and developmental level of the person. One of the challenges of implementing traditional therapy with individuals with dual diagnoses is that the structure of traditional mental health settings can create additional barriers. This chapter will discuss those challenges as well as adaptations to the settings. In addition, Appendix C provides activities and lessons that have been adapted for use with people who have dual diagnoses.

Inpatient Treatment Setting

The structure of an inpatient treatment setting, such as a psychiatric hospital, from the beginning creates complications for an individual with an intellectual disability. First, the intake is predominantly a session of verbal questions the person is asked to answer. This can be really difficult for a person for whom verbal communication is not a strength. In addition, gathering history is difficult because the person often does not know all of the information, resulting in the setting having limited background information. When the person is brought to the unit, there is typically not a lot of introduction to the setting and what to expect while there. In addition, the daily schedule is usually in writing. This can be difficult for the person to follow. It is also often not clear who their contact person is if they need something.

During a person's stay at the hospital there are typically a lot of group therapy sessions. These sessions are presented verbally. Verbal skills and receptive language can be barriers to the person's participation in these groups. In addition, much of the therapy is insight-oriented or teaching skills to be used independently, which is challenging for a person with an intellectual disability. Coping with the mental health issue independently requires executive functioning, a known weakness for individuals with an intellectual disability. There is not a lot of peer interaction so often the person approaches nurses and staff when looking to engage with someone. There is also a lot of unstructured time, which is very difficult for this population. For these reasons, nurses and staff can get frustrated with the level of need that individuals with dual diagnoses often require. These frustrations can lead to assumptions that the challenges are "behavioral" and not related to mental health.

Upon discharge there are further complications. The skills taught during the person's stay are meant to be used independently. There is often not a lot of communication with outside support people about what was focused on during the person's stay. The person is often not able to tell care providers what occurred there and what follow-up support would be needed. The focus of the mental health system is to help the person become safe so he or she can be discharged back into the home setting, but individuals with dual diagnoses are likely to need follow-up support (often intensive support) to continue their progress. To help facilitate the success and progress for a person during an inpatient stay the following recommendations are provided:

- Encourage a support staff from the person's community setting to accompany him or her to the intake to provide history and relevant information. This can be important as it relates to the person's likes and dislikes. It can also prevent a lot of stress if things are shared about what is upsetting for that person. For example, if the person is afraid of needles or needs physical distance between him and others it is important information to share. Alternatively, it is important at that time to share activities that the person finds calming, such as listening to music or looking at a magazine.

• Introduce to the individual a nurse or contact person who is available to answer questions or discuss concerns. In addition, as each shift changes the new contact person should introduce himself or herself to the individual.

• Provide a tour of the unit. This should include showing the person where the T.V. room and access to activities are located, such as games and books.

• Introduce the individual to his or her roommate. It may even help to begin a conversation between the person and the roommate before leaving the room.

• Check in with the person at least every ten minutes after first arriving. This should not be time-consuming. It could consist of just saying "hello" and observing the person's level of comfort in the milieu or could include a short conversation.

• Provide a picture schedule so the person knows where to go and what groups are being offered. This schedule can be as simple as a handwritten schedule with simple drawings to represent the activities. It can also be more complex and include pictures from clip art programs. Included on the schedule should be wake-up and bedtimes, mealtimes, free time and group time. If there are any particular groups the staff believe would be beneficial for the person, they should be highlighted so the individual doesn't forget.

• Provide therapy and skills that are visual and experiential (sample groups are provided in Appendix C of this book).

• Provide a list of activities (in picture form if needed) the person can participate in during the unstructured time. The person may need help getting started with an activity. For example, if doing a puzzle, the individual may need help finding a place to do it and help setting it up.

• Introduce the nurse or staff member who is available to the person each time there is a shift change.

Outpatient Treatment Setting

Many of the therapeutic complications in an inpatient setting are similar to an outpatient setting. The most challenging is developing ways to present the information so that the person can generalize them to outside of the office. Again, visual and experiential strategies are the best. Any of the group training activities provided in Appendix

C can be easily adapted to individual therapy as well.

In an outpatient setting it is important to involve the support people in the person's life. The support person can be a great source of information for how the person is doing at home, whether they are using the skills being taught, and offering suggestions about areas of focus. Together they can develop ways the support team can assist the person. This can include coaching and support of the skills being taught in sessions. That said, this should only be done with the permission of the person.

A great model of adapting a traditional therapy and using support staff as home coaches is the Skills System developed by Julie Brown (2011). The Skills System adapted some concepts from Dialectical Behavior Therapy (Linehan, 1993) to be used with adults with dual diagnoses. She integrated visual aids and concrete concepts to develop skills to cope with emotional dysregulation. Included in her program is a weekly group and individual therapy session for the person and a monthly training for the care providers to learn the skills. The monthly training offers guidance on how to support the person in using the skills at home.

The Wellness Recovery Action Plan developed by Mary Ellen Copeland (2002) is a tool used in the mental health system to monitor symptoms and develop a plan to reduce those symptoms. It is a system that has been introduced to people with dual diagnoses and has been an effective tool. It is a treatment plan that is written by the individual, with the help of care providers when needed. Because it is a written plan (picture icons can also be used), it addresses the strength of visual cues in treatment planning. In addition, it is the property of the person, which allows the person to feel as though he or she has an active part in the behavioral support system. The WRAP has several purposes when considering the cognitive and emotional issues common for people with dual diagnoses.

- It can help the person feel ownership over treatment and feel empowered to make changes. It is his or her plan and the information written in the plan is what the person has chosen to include. This is different than other treatment plans that may have been written for the person by others.
- It can provide a system of communication across settings (group home to hospital to day program to job). The person may choose to share the information with others in order to receive similar support in multiple settings. It also offers a

place to add things from different settings that may help at home. For example, if a job coach identifies a coping skill, the coach can help the person write it in the plan. That way the home staff can use this effective strategy as well.

- It can be used as a resource for the individual for effective coping strategies. It is great to provide a list of new options the person can learn when the strategies that have been identified are not effective.

- It can be used as a reminder of the treatment plan they have decided upon (it is visual, reminds them of options and is personal). Oftentimes, when a person is feeling overwhelmed it is difficult to remember the strategies that have been learned. This a great tool to provide visual reminders of those strategies.

- It can be used as a form to communicate to others who their preferred support people are in times of crisis. In the plan, the person chooses from a list of preferred and non-preferred people to help when a crisis arises. This can be a powerful tool and communicates to the individual that his or her choices are important, even in times when others are making decisions for that person.

- It can be a guide to past and present medications. In addition to current medication, the plan includes past medications and the reason they are no longer prescribed.

- It includes a list of support people who can provide information to hospitals (history, behavioral pattern, helpful interventions, etc.).

Additional Clinical Interventions

Because of the complexities of working with this population, professionals and care providers are required to have knowledge and expertise in developmental disorders, intellectual disability, and psychiatric disorders. For this reason, additional training is often needed to support the team. Some training outlines are provided in Appendix B that include training for care providers, hospital staff, and residential staff. A variety of therapy group trainings and activities can be found in Appendix C of this manual including training in relaxation skills, boundary trainings for effective relationships, the development of work readiness skills, and money management. Any of the therapy group exercises can be easily adapted as individual therapy and coaching tools.

Chapter 10

Putting it All Together:
A Step-By-Step Approach

Identifying the cause of a behavioral challenge requires attention to detail. It involves detective work and the ability to stand back with enough objectivity to decipher the clues. The following are real stories of individuals who presented with behavioral problems. Each story is followed by an analysis using the hierarchy discussed in the previous chapters. Initially, medical causes are ruled out. This is followed by a rule out of psychiatric conditions. It is important to consider how the intellectual disability is interfacing with the psychiatric issues. Finally, consideration is given as to whether or not the challenging behavior is a learned behavior. Sometimes the behavior is the result of all of these factors combined, including medical, psychiatric, and behavioral contributors.

The Story of Anna

Anna was a 35-year-old Caucasian woman who lived in an adult residential facility. The home had five other residents. She had lived there for five years. She had a history of self-injurious behavior which involved picking her skin. Typically, this behavior had been localized to her arms. On occasion, the behavior resulted in open wounds, but incidents of skin picking had significantly decreased in the past several years. Within the span of a few weeks, the behavior significantly increased in not only frequency, but intensity. It had increased to the extent that behavioral consultation services were requested because of how raw her skin had become. Anna had begun picking at her knees, her hands, as well as her arms, which was a change in her usual presentation of the behavior. Incidents of skin picking were now accompanied by agitation, including pacing, difficulty sitting still, decreased attention span, and insomnia. Previously, episodes of skin picking were not accompanied by such restlessness. Anna was non-verbal and she was diagnosed with Severe Intellectual Disability and Obsessive-Compulsive Disorder. She was not taking any psychotropic medications.

Step 1 – Rule-out the medical causes or contributors. Information was obtained on her current and past medical conditions. No skin conditions were identified. She did not have a history of any skin conditions, such as eczema, which can reoccur. There were no recent changes in medications that may have resulted in an allergic reaction. However, she had not seen a physician or dermatologist to ensure that a medical condition was not causing or contributing to the behavior.

Step 2 – Consider psychiatric causes. Although medical causes had not yet been ruled out, possible psychiatric conditions were also being considered since she was diagnosed with Obsessive-Compulsive Disorder. The incidents of skin picking could be attributed to this condition. However, the severity and frequency of her picking at her skin significantly increased in a short span of time and deviated from the usual presentation of being contained to just her arms. There were also changes in her sleep pattern which coincided with the re-emergence of skin picking. She had not experienced any difficulties with sleeping previously. She had no history of insomnia or any sleep disturbance.

According to the *Diagnostic and Statistical Manual of Mental Disorders – Fourth Edition- Text Revision,* the possible psychiatric disorders which could fit this presentation would be Obsessive-Compulsive Disorder (OCD) or Impulse Control Disorder, NOS. The diagnosis of OCD could account for the increase in the behavior because OCD symptoms can wax and wane and flare-up during times of stress. It could have interfered with her sleep if the urges to pick increased. However, the diagnosis did not fully describe all of the accompanying behaviors, such as her difficulty sitting still and her shortened attention span. Therefore, it would seem that some other factors or variables were operating or influencing the behavior.

Step 3 – Rule-out the behavioral causes. Was her behavior a learned behavior and if so, what influences could possibly have been maintaining the behavior? A functional analysis was completed and it was discovered that this behavior was occurring throughout the day and in all situations, but it was particularly intense at night while she was in her bed. Any changes that had occurred in her life or environment were explored. The only change that had been introduced was a change in bedrooms because another resident had moved out of the home. After the individual left, Anna had moved into her bedroom because it was larger. No other changes could be indentified either in the individuals who helped care for her, or in her environment. Further observations and meetings with Anna occurred, and upon closer observation it was noted that she didn't seem to be picking at her skin as much as she was scratching it.

The Final Analysis. This is where the results of the detective work came together. All of the information gained from reviewing the categories in Chapter 4 and Chapter 5 helped provide information as to whether or not the behavior could be attributed to medical, psychiatric, or behavioral reasons. Since she had not seen a dermatologist or her family practice physician, the medical rule-outs had not yet been addressed. Staff had only her past medical history and her current medical conditions which could not account for the increase in skin picking. The behavior was occurring across environments and with different people, but it was particularly intense at night while in her bedroom. The onset of the significant increase in the behavior had been rather sudden and the behavior didn't exactly look like her behavior of compulsively picking at her skin, although it was initially labeled as an increase in skin picking. There had also been the recent change in her sleeping patterns. She was no longer sleeping through the night. She would wake up several times throughout the night and pick at her skin.

The only changes in her life had been the fact that she changed rooms and another resident moved out of the home. When she changed rooms, she was given a different mattress that had been donated because the other resident took the mattress Anna had been using.

Given the sudden increase in her behavior, the change in her sleep patterns, and changes in the description of the behavior, without any significant changes in her life circumstances, the possibility of an underlying medical cause was further explored. Anna was taken to the dermatologist and diagnosed with scabies, which she apparently caught from the donated mattress. The mattress had been infected. The behavior was not one of compulsive skin picking, but she was actually scratching due to the intense itching caused by the scabies.

The scabies was treated and her skin healed. Occasionally, she would still pick at her skin, but not to the degree that she had been doing.

Several important lessons can be learned from working with Anna. It is important not to assume anything when presented with behavioral challenges. It would have been easy to attribute the increase of picking behaviors to her diagnosis of Obsessive-Compulsive Disorder (OCD) without looking any further. After all, she had been exhibiting this behavior for years and symptoms of OCD can wax and wane. However, once the hierarchy was used which consisted of ruling out any medical causes, ruling out a psychiatric disorder, and ruling out learned behaviors, the cause was identified. It highlights the need to "go back to basics" and consider the hierarchy in trying to determine the cause of a behavioral problem. Start from the beginning. Don't assume anything, and be attentive to the details, and to subtle changes.

The Story of Dee

Dee was a 50-year-old woman who had a long-standing drug and alcohol abuse history, as well as a history of hospitalizations for suicidal ideation, depression, anxiety, auditory hallucinations, and violent behavior. Over the years she had carried the diagnoses of Paranoid Schizophrenia, Moderate Intellectual Disability, and Mild Intellectual Disability. Dee tested positive for multiple drugs when she was born. She lived at home until she was nine-years-old at which time her family sought assistance in finding an out-of-home placement because she was becoming aggressive towards other children and adults. She then was in and out of various homes throughout her childhood, such as foster homes and group homes, until she ultimately lived on the streets. She attempted to live in several group homes as an adult, however, her preference was to be with her "street family." Partly, there was the connection with the other homeless people she knew, however, there was also a significant substance abuse problem. Dee had used drugs most of her adult life with very limited periods of sobriety.

At the time behavioral consultation was requested, Dee was getting out of jail on a drug possession charge. She was being released to a Sober Living Home and was required to check in with her probation officer daily and complete random drug tests.

Step 1 – Rule-out medical causes or contributors. Dee had a seizure disorder, which was controlled by anti-convulsant medication. She had not had a seizure in at least three years. At one time she also used a CPAP machine for sleep apnea. Dee said that the machine never worked correctly and that she stopped using it. Sleep apnea can have a significant impact on a person's level of fatigue, which in turn can increase feelings of anxiety and depression. Because she was homeless much of the time, sleep was likely to be regularly disrupted anyway. This, paired with the identified sleep apnea, made her even more vulnerable to decreased frustration tolerance and agitation that can accompany sleep deprivation.

Dee was taking Dilantin to control her seizures. She was also taking Seroquel and Geodon for psychosis, with Cogentin to address the side effects. Dee voluntarily was taking the injectable medication, Prolixin, which is another anti-psychotic medication. There were concerns about the fact that she was taking three different anti-psychotic medications. In addition, she was receiving an injectable medication because of the challenge of taking it regularly when she was homeless. That also meant that it was likely that she was taking the other medication inconsistently. In addition, an important consideration was the interaction her drug and alcohol use had with her medication. The true effectiveness of her medication was unknown. She did not keep regular psychiatric appointments. She took her medication inconsistently, and her drug use was likely to have a significant impact.

Step 2 – Consider psychiatric causes. The most prominent challenge for Dee was her long-standing drug use. She had very limited periods of time when she has been free of drug use, despite some participation in drug programs. Her addiction was a strong force that challenged her on a daily basis. When she was living in group homes she had frequent episodes of leaving without telling anyone. This resulted in either her being discharged because they couldn't monitor her safety, or her becoming angry and quitting the program.

Dee carried a diagnosis of Paranoid Schizophrenia, however, it was also known that she had been using drugs since her teens. Whether the reported auditory hallucinations were the result of her long-standing drug use or a predisposition to a psychotic disorder was unknown.

Dee had periods of depression and anxiety. Given her history of out-of-home placements, problems with the law, and hospitalizations, it was important to assess the extent she was also depressed. It may be that she was using substances as a self-medicating tool when she was feeling depressed or anxious. It may also have been a way that she felt connected to her "family on the streets."

Step 3 – Rule-out behavioral causes (i.e., learned behaviors). When living in the group homes the main focus was on her level of agitation and anger, as well as her frequent attempts to leave the facility to use drugs. While the homes brought her to AA meetings and she attended some outpatient drug treatment programs, the homes were not integrating support for her around her addiction. In the homes they were focused on the "behavior." For many drug users, their moods become agitated and they can become explosive as the result of the drug use. If they have not used in awhile and are craving the drug, they are often agitated and angry. In addition, while the influence of those she knew on the streets at times encouraged drug use and illegal activity, she described them as her family. She felt very close to them. When feeling alone, depressed, agitated, or depressed she sought the comfort of those who knew her best.

A questionnaire completed by one of the group facilitators and her group home administrator revealed that one of the things that was most motivating for Dee was a very high desire to learn. Individuals with the same profile were motivated by exploring new places and trying new things. This was important because it meant that she was more likely to seek out stimulating environments if she felt bored.

It was noted upon meeting Dee that she had significant difficulty with receptive language. She was fluently verbal, therefore, it was assumed by most who worked with her that she understood and remembered the things that they spoke about. This was likely one reason the substance abuse programs were not effective for her.

The Final Analysis. Dee's story is the perfect example of the importance of integrating interventions that address both the developmental disorder as well as the psychiatric issues. Just addressing the substance abuse and psychiatric issues were not effective because of the cognitive complications of the developmental disorder. She had tremendous difficulty following the discussions in the groups and when asked about them later did not remember the topics or skills taught. In addition, just addressing the behavioral challenges was not effective because her substance use was such a driving force. In summary, she did not improve when she was living in group homes for people with developmental disorders. In addition, she did not improve when she was participating in general substance abuse programs. She needed both.

The team developed various wrap-around supports for her. She lived in a group home with a low staff to resident ratio so that she could participate in a lot of activities that she found fun and met her need for curiosity. The staff were also trained to address the substance abuse issue consistently and frequently throughout the day using Wow Papers, certificates, and helping her identify the need to attend an NA group. The staff also received training on the importance of her participating in a substance abuse treatment day program and making her appointments with the probation officer. In addition, the substance abuse program staff were trained in communicating with a person with an intellectual disability. This included using visual examples and drawings. It also included teaching them ways to communicate verbally in a manner that did not include too much content at once, focusing on one goal at a time, and presenting the same goal in multiple ways. Lastly, the substance abuse day program had a psychiatrist on staff who could monitor her medication. In addition, the group home was to follow-up on a sleep study to address the current status of her sleep apnea.

The Story of Peter

Peter was a 42-year-old male who lived in an adult residential facility. He was diagnosed with Mild Intellectual Disability. He had lived at home for many years but after his parents passed away he went to live in an adult residential facility with several other people who had an intellectual disability. The home closed after several years and he moved to another facility. He came to the attention of a behavior specialist hired by an agency because of the numerous behavioral challenges he was exhibiting in the home. He had been living in the home for several years but his behavioral challenges kept increasing. He was having incidents of aggression towards staff and incidents of defecating in his pants even though he was capable of using the bathroom on his own. He frequently complained about problems in his life and he was very talkative with the staff, often repeating the same questions. Staff described him as being very needy for their attention and manipulative. As a result, staff who worked closely with him began getting easily irritated with his behaviors and feeling burned out.

Step 1 – Rule-out the medical. Peter presented with several behavioral problems including aggression, intermittent incontinence, running away, and frequently repeating himself. It was important to separately review the behaviors and use the hierarchy to decipher the cause of each of the behaviors. The easiest behavior to begin with was the incontinence and to consider its possible medical causes or contributors. Although he had a physical in the past year, the issue of incontinence was not specifically brought to the attention of his physician. In preparation for the visit to the doctor, information was obtained about the frequency of the incontinence, and the circumstances under which it occurred, along with the history, including how long it had been occurring. His medications and diet were also reviewed with his physician. The medical appointment resulted in a diagnosis of constipation with overflow incontinence. As a result, he was prescribed a stool softener and no further problems were reported. Consequently, the issue was resolved at the initial level of exploration.

Step 2 – Consider psychiatric causes. The behavior of him frequently repeating himself was considered in light of possible medical causes. It raised the question of whether or not he was suffering from memory problems which may have an underlying physical cause. Since the result of his most recent physical examination and consultation indicated he was in good health with the exception of periodic bouts of constipation, psychiatric rule-outs were considered. Upon further exploration of the exact content and frequency of him repeating himself, it was discovered that the content of his conversations and his repetitiveness often focused on specific worries that he had regarding several areas of his life. He would frequently bring up the same topics, such as concerns about his sister and her health, worries about his money, and worries about interpersonal problems he had at the day program.

Upon further discussion with his sister, information was obtained regarding his family's psychiatric history. He had two sisters who suffered from anxiety disorders and his current symptoms could meet the diagnostic criteria for a Generalized Anxiety Disorder. This disorder is an anxiety condition in which an individual worries about several areas of his life and these worries are out of proportion to the situation. The worries also interfere with the individual's life. Therefore, Peter's repetitive questioning may have been misinterpreted by the staff as attention-seeking behavior but appeared to be more reflective of his anxiety and his tendency to worry too much. It was also discovered by talking with his sister and reviewing his records that he had a trauma history. He witnessed his father hitting his mother when he was a child and an adolescent. He also was a victim of physical abuse by his father on numerous occasions. His trauma history had implications for his current relationships and the attachments he formed. If staff became irritated with his extensive worries and his repeatedly talking about the same issues, this caused him more anxiety given his abuse background.

Step 3 – Rule-out behavioral causes (i.e., learned behaviors). Although Peter's behavior of frequently talking about the same topics and repeating himself could be explained at the second level of analysis (i.e., an anxiety disorder), it could also have a learned component. By repeatedly going to staff and talking about his worries, he would frequently get attention and reassurance which could help to maintain the behavior.

When considering his aggressive behavior, the treatment of aggression necessitates a comprehensive assessment, since there are many potential causes of aggression. Aggression can be the result of a medical illness or it can also be a feature of a psychiatric condition such as a mood disorder or impulse control disorder. In consultation with Peter's physician, no medical cause could be identified that could account for his aggressive incidents. The second step of the analysis involved considering psychiatric conditions as a possible cause. Aggression can be a feature of several different psychiatric conditions or it can be the central component of a psychiatric condition. Aggression may also be a purposeful behavior or a reaction to an environmental stressor. An individual may become aggressive as a way to avoid a task, escape from a task, communicate frustration, or use it as a means to obtain a goal or discharge tension.

In this particular situation, a functional analysis of Peter's aggression was conducted, which examined the "who, what, where, and when" around the occurrence of aggression. This type of analysis revealed it occurred in two types of circumstances. When staff became frustrated with him over his worries and frequent questioning, they would respond with irritation. This triggered a level of increased of physical tension and anxiety in him based on his trauma history. In addition, he observed his father hitting his mother on numerous occasions and his father was able to get what he wanted by intimidating his mother. Consequently, there was also a learned element to Peter's aggression based on the role modeling he observed.

The Final Analysis. After reviewing all of the behaviors from the three step analysis or hierarchy, a treatment plan was developed. This included addressing the elements of his behaviors which had a medical cause, along with addressing the psychiatric and learned elements of the behavioral challenges. To address the encopresis, a stool softener was added to treat the constipation with overflow incontinence. He was also encouraged to drink more fluids.

Both cognitive and behavioral interventions were also devised to address his excessive worries and ruminations which would also aggravate the staff. These techniques included instructions in relaxation techniques such as breathing exercises, progressive muscle relaxation exercises, and visual imagery for relaxation. In addition, distraction techniques were used to refocus his energies. Established times were set in which he could talk about his worries to the staff (i.e., a stimulus control procedure) and staff would also help him to problem-solve or work on surrender skills if he couldn't control a situation. Staff was also encouraged to provide him with a high level of attention when the content of his conversations did not involve topics of worry. Staff was also informed of Peter's traumatic history while living at home and how important it was to maintain a calm demeanor and not show irritation, given the history of abuse he suffered from his father. This helped to lower his level of anxiety. Anger management strategies were also introduced to help Peter calm down when he did not get his way in a situation. Staff also ensured that any aggressive behavior he exhibited was not rewarded by allowing him to escape a situation or obtain a desired item through intimidation.

The interventions for Peter required the identification and appreciation of all the factors, including the medical, psychiatric, and learning histories, which can influence behavior or cause the behavioral challenges. To attribute the behaviors to only attention-seeking or manipulative motives, which may occur among this population, is an oversimplification of the complexities of human behavior and a disservice to those individuals with an intellectual disability.

If each of these steps in the assessment process are not considered, you have not reached the final analysis. Assumptions and rash conclusions can cause continued distress for the person. Imagine if the three individuals described were never offered the life of dignity that they achieved: Anna continued to suffer from scabies, Dee continued to go from program to program because no one place met all of her needs, and Peter's physical and emotional needs were never considered and the assumption remained that it was all "behavioral." In the final analysis, assume nothing, observe closely, and take the time to do the research. Most importantly, appreciate the unique expressions of the psychiatric, medical, and psychological needs of the individuals with an intellectual disability and be wiser from their teachings.

References

Aman, M. & Singh, N. (1986). *The aberrant behavior checklist.* East Aurora, New York: Slosson Educational Publications, Inc.

American Psychiatric Association (2000). *Diagnostic and statistical manual of mental disorders* (4th ed., Text Revision). Washington, D.C.: Author.

Benbadis, S. & Heriaud, L. (2002). Comphrensive Epilepsy Program. Retrieved on line on 5/2211 from http://hsc.usf.edu/COM/epilepsy/PNES_USF.html

Bosch, J.J. (2003). Health maintenance throughout the life span for the individual with Down syndrome. *Journal of the American Academy of Nurse Practitioners, 15*(1), 5-17.

Brown, J.F. (2011) *The skills system instructor's guide: An emotion-regulation skills curriculum for all learning abilities.* Bloomington, IN: iUniverse.

Budman, C.L., Bruun, R., Park, K.S., Lesser, M., & Olson, M. (2000). Explosive outbursts in children with Tourette's disorder. *Journal of the American Academy of Child and Adolescent Psychiatry, 39(10),* 1270-1276

Chaplin, J. P. & Krawiec, T. S. (1974). *Systems and theories of psychology* (3rd ed.). New York: Holt, Rinehart, & Winston Inc.

Charlot, L., Fox, S., Silka, V.R., Hurley, A., Lowry, M.A., & Pary, R. (2007). Mood disorders. In R. Fletcher, E. Loschen, C. Stavrakaki, & M. First, (Eds.), *Diagnostic manual – Intellectual disability (DM-ID): A clinical guide for diagnosis of mental disorders in persons with intellectual disability* (pp. 157-186). Kingston, NY: NADD Press.

Copeland, M.E. (2002). *Wellness recovery action plan.* Dummerson, VT: Peach Press.

Dana, L. (1993). Personality disorders in persons with mental retardation: assessment and diagnosis. In R.J. Fletcher & A. Dosen (Eds.), *Mental health aspects of mental retardation: Progress in assessment and treatment.* New York: Lexington Books.

DeLeon, I.S., Uy, M., & Gutshall, K. (2005). Noncontingent reinforcement and competing stimuli in the treatment of pseudoseizures and destructive behaviors. *Behavior Intervention, 20,* 203-217.

DeVeer, A.J.E., Bos, J.T., Niezen-de Boer, R.C., Bohmer, C.J.M., & Francke, A.L. (2008). The symptoms of gastroesophageal reflux disease in severely mentally retarded people: A systematic review, *Gastroenterology, 8*(23). Retrieved from http://creative commons.orglicenses/by/2.0)

Espie, C.A. (2000). Sleep and disorders of sleep in people with mental retardation. *Current Opinion in Psychiatry, 13,* 507-511.

Favilla, M., & Mucci, M. (2000). Generalized anxiety disorders in adolescents and young adults with mild mental retardation. *Psychiatry, 63*(1): 54-64.

Feinstein, R., & Reiss, A.L. (1996). Psychiatric disorder in mentally retarded children and adolescents: the challenging of meaningful diagnosis. *Child and Adolescent Psychiatric Clinic of North America, 5,* 827-852.

Ferguson, M. (1980). *The Aquarian conspiracy.* Los Angeles: Tarcher.

First, M.B., & Tasman, A. (2004). *DSM-IV-TR mental disorders: Diagnosis, etiology, and treatment.* West Sussex, England: John Wiley & Sons, Ltd.

Fletcher, R., Loschen, E., Stavrakaki, C., & First, M. (2007a). *Diagnostic manual-intellectual disability (DM-ID). A clinical guide for diagnosis of mental disorders in persons with intellectual disability.* Kingston, NY: NADD Press.

Fletcher, R., Loschen, E., Stavrakaki, C., & First, M. (2007b). *Diagnostic manual-intellectual disability (DM-ID). A textbook of mental disorders in persons with intellectual disability.* Kingston, NY: NADD Press.

Fuller, M. A. & Sajavoeic, M. (2002). *Psychotropic drug information handbook* (3rd ed.). Hudson, OH: Lexi-Comp, Inc.

Gedye, A. (1992). Recognizing obsessive-compulsive disorder in clients with developmental disabilities. *The Habilitative Mental Healthcare Newsletter 11,* (11), p. 73-77.

Griffiths, D. M., Stavrakkaki, C., & Summers, J. (2002). *Dual diagnosis: An introduction to the mental health needs of persons with developmental disabilities.* Ontario, Canada: Habilitative Mental Health Resource Network.

Holmes, T.H., & Rahe, R.H., (1967). The social adjustment rating scale. *Journal of Psychosomatic Research, 11,* 213.

Homatidis, S. (2005). Challenges in identifying mental health issues in individuals with severe autism. *Journal on Developmental Disabilities, 9(2),* 55-59.

Iwata, B.A., Dorsey, M.F., Slifer, K.J., Bauman, K.E., & Richman, G.S. (1982). Toward a functional analysis of self-injury. *Analysis and Intervention in Developmental Disabilities, 2, 3-20.*

King. B. (May, 2006). Medications simplified: A walk through what to choose for whom and for what, when? A paper presented at *Innovative Approaches: Treatment for People with Developmental Disabilities and Psychiatric Disorders.* Ontario, CA.

Levitas, A. (1997). Laws of pharmacology. *The Habilitative Mental Healthcare Newsletter,* 16(4), 67-69.

Levitas, A. Dykens, E., Finucane, B., Kates, W.R. (2007a). Behavioral phenotype of genetic disorders. In R. Fletcher, E. Loschen, C. Stavrakaki, & M. First, (Eds.), *Diagnostic manual – Intellectual disability (DM-ID): A clinical guide for diagnosis of mental disorders in persons with intellectual disability* (pp. 25-50). Kingston, NY: NADD Press.

Levitas, A. Dykens, E., Finucane, B., Kates, W.R. (2007b). Behavioral phenotype of genetic disorders. In R. Fletcher, E. Loschen, C. Stavrakaki, & M. First, (Eds.), *Diagnostic manual – Intellectual disability (DM-ID): A textbook of diagnosis of mental disorders in persons with intellectual disability* (pp. 33-62). Kingston, NY: NADD Press.

Levitas, A. & Hurley, A.D. (2007). Adjustment disorders. In R. Fletcher, E. Loschen, C. Stavrakaki, & M. First, (Eds.), *Diagnostic manual – Intellectual disability: A textbook of diagnosis of mental disorders in persons with intellectual disability.* Kingston, NY: NADD Press.

Lindsay, W.R., Dana, L.A., Dosen, A., Gabriel, S.R., & Young, S. (2007). Personality disorders. In R. Fletcher, E. Loschen, C. Stavrakaki, & M. First, (Eds.), *Diagnostic manual – Intellectual disability (DM-ID): A clinical guide for diagnosis of mental disorders in persons with intellectual disability* (pp. 157-186). Kingston, NY: NADD Press.

Linehan, Marsha (1993). *Skills training manual for treating Borderline Personality Disorder.* New York: Guilford Press.

Matson, J.L. (1995). *The Diagnostic Assessment for the Severely Handicapped –II.* Baton Rouge, LA: Scientific Publishers, Inc.

Moss, S.C., Prosser, H., Costello, H., Simpson, N., Patel, P., Rowe, S., . . . Hatton, C. (1998). Reliability and validity of the PAS-ADD Checklist for detecting psychiatric disorders in adults with intellectual disability. *Journal of Intellectual Disability Research, 42,* 173-183.

Neppe, V.M., & Tucker, G.J. (1988). Modern perspectives on epilepsy in relation to psychiatry; classification and evaluation. *Hosp Community Psychiatry. 39*(3), 263-271.

Nugent, J.A. (1997). *Handbook on dual diagnosis: supporting people with a developmental disability and a mental health problem.* Self: Nugent Training and Consulting Services: Author.

Personality Psychology. (n.d.). In *Wikipedia.* Retrieved August 22, 2010 from http://en.wikipedia.org/wiki/Personality psychology

Reiss, S. (1988). *Reiss screen for maladaptive behaviours.* Ohio: International Diagnostic Systems, Inc.

Reiss, S. (1990). Prevalence of dual diagnoses in community-based day programs in the Chicago metropolitan area. *American Journal of Mental Retardation, 94,* 578-585.

Reiss, S. (2001). *Reiss profile of fundamental goals and motivation sensitivities for persons with mental retardation.*

Reiss, S., Goldberg, B., & Ryan, R. (1993). Questions and answers on mental illness in persons with mental retardation. The Arc/United States Web site: http://www.thearc.org.

Reiss, S., Leviton, G.W., & Szyszko, J. (1982). Emotional disturbance and mental retardation: diagnostic overshadowing. *American Journal of Mental Deficiency, 86,* 567-574.

Richdale, A.L., Cotton, S., & Hibbit, K. (1999). Sleep and behavior disturbance in Prader-Willi syndrome: A questionnaire study. *Journal of Intellectual Disabilities Research, 43,* 380-392.

Rifkin, A., & Barnhill, L.J. (2007). Impulses-control disorders not elsewhere classified. In R. Fletcher, E. Loschen, C. Stavrakaki, & M. First, (Eds.), *Diagnostic manual – Intellectual disability (DM-ID): A clinical guide for diagnosis of mental disorders in persons with intellectual disability* (pp. 291-300). Kingston, NY: NADD Press.

Ryan, R.M. (1996). *Handbook of mental health care for persons with developmental disabilities.* Denver, CO: S&B Publishing.

Ryan, R.M. (2001). Recognizing psychosis in nonverbal patients with developmental disabilities. *Psychiatric Times,* 18 (12).

Seyle, H. (1974). *Stress without distress.* Philadelphia: Lippincott.

Skinner, B.F. (1953). *Science and human behavior.* New York: Macmillan.

Sobsey, D. (1994). *Violence and abuse in the lives of people with disabilities: The end of silent acceptance?* Baltimore: P.H. Brookes Publishing Co.

Sovner, R., Beasley, J., & Desnoyers Hurley, A. (1995). How long should a psychiatric inpatient stay be for a person with developmental disabilities? *Habilitative Mental Healthcare Newsletter, 14*(1), 1-8.

Sovner, R., & DesMoyers Hurley, A. (1986). Four factors affecting the diagnosis of psychiatric disorders in mentally retarded persons. *Psychiatric Aspects of Mental Retardation Reviews,* 5, 45-49.

Stiefel, Scott (2007). *Developmental Disabilities and Sleep: Disorders Not Recognized and Not Treated.* Paper presented at Developmental Disabilities Nurses Association.

Stray-Gundersen, K. (1995). *Babies with Down syndrome: A new parents' guide* (2nd ed.). Bethesda, MD: Woodbine House.

Szymanski, L., & King, B. (1999). *Summary of the practice parameters for the assessment and treatment of children, adolescents, and adults with mental retardation and comorbid mental disorders.* AACAP Publications

Department, Washington, D.C. Retrieved from http://www.aacap. org/clinical/parameters/summaries/mr.htm

Thorndike, E.L. (1911). *Animal intelligence: Experimental studies.* New York: Macmillan.

Vgontzas, A. N. & Kales, A. (1999). Sleep and its disorders. *Annual Review of Medicine, 50,* 387-400.

White, R.S. (1998). DMR Medical Advisory #98-5: Standards for multiple drug use. http://www.dmr.state.ct.us/publications/ centralofc/hcs ma98-5.htm.

Zwakhalen, S., Van Dongen, K., Hamers, J., & Abu-Sadd, H.H. (2004). Pain assessment in intellectually disabled people: nonverbal indicators. *Journal of Advanced Nursing, 45(3),* 236-245.

Appendix A

Diagnosis and Treatment
of Aggression

Chronic and severe aggression can lead to a psychiatric hospitalization or an admission to a more restrictive setting for an individual with an intellectual disability. It is a common complaint presented to psychiatrists, psychologists, and behavior specialists who work with this population. To provide effective treatment, a comprehensive evaluation is required since there are many potential causes of aggression. Aggression can be an associated symptom of a primary psychiatric condition or it can be the result of an underlying medical issue. It can also be a purposeful or learned behavior. The following are some potential causes of aggression:

1. **Aggression and Psychiatric Disorders.** Aggression can be a feature of any of the following psychiatric conditions:
   - Substance Use – It can occur as a result of intoxication or withdrawal.
   - Schizophrenia – Impulsive aggression can be an associated feature and occur in response to delusions and hallucinations.
   - Obsessive-Compulsive Disorder – Impulsive aggression can also appear as a variant of OCD.
   - Mood Disorder – Aggression can occur during a manic episode.
   - Depressive Disorder – Aggression can occur in response to increasing irritability.
   - Anxiety Disorder – Aggression can occur in response to increasing anxiety.
   - Tourette's disorder – Individuals with Tourette's disorder can be prone to rage reactions as a result of an underlying dysregulation of the nervous system (Budman et al. 2000).

- Posttraumatic Stress Disorder – Outbursts of anger which can escalate into aggression can occur as a result of increased arousal.
- Intermittent Explosive Disorder – Impulsive aggression can be a central feature and can be preceded by a period of increasing tension and arousal.
- Borderline Personality Disorder – Aggression can occur due to periods of intense anger and difficulties controlling anger which can be a symptom of this disorder.
- Antisocial Personality Disorder – Impulsive aggression can be a central feature of this disorder and can be preceded by a period of increasing tension and arousal.

Aggression can emerge during the course of a psychiatric illness or it can be the central component of the condition. According to Ruth Ryan (1996), the most common psychiatric conditions associated with violent behavior among individuals with an intellectual disability who were treated at her clinic included anxiety disorders, particularly posttraumatic stress reactions, panic attacks, and generalized anxiety. She also found aggression to occur among individuals who were depressed or in a manic phase of a bipolar disorder.

Psychosis and aggression. Aggression which results from schizophrenia may occur in response to the delusions or hallucinations that the individual is experiencing. The person may become violent as a result of command hallucinations or in response to the feelings associated with the delusional beliefs.

Childhood disorders and aggression. Chronic aggression, along with chronic impulsivity, may be part of a diagnosis first identified during childhood or adolescence, such as a Conduct Disorder or Attention Deficit Hyperactivity Disorder.

Autism and aggression. Aggression may be present among individuals with autistic spectrum disorders. Aggression may be triggered by exposure to highly stimulating and noisy environments. Individuals with autism may also become aggressive when presented with changes in their routine or in response to transitions. Their deficits with cognitive flexibility can make it difficult for them to make the cognitive shifts involved in transitioning from one task to another. Consequently, they may respond with a rigid adherence to sameness in their lives. Changes in a routine can serve as an antecedent for aggression. They may also respond aggressively when demands are placed on them. Individuals whose diagnoses are within the autism spectrum can show great variability in the frequency and intensity of their aggression across environments.

Obsessive-Compulsive Disorder and aggression. Aggression may occur among individuals with intellectual disability who also have Obsessive-Compulsive Disorder when their rituals are interrupted. Individuals who support them may be unaware of these rituals. For example, an individual who is non-verbal and is cognitively functioning within the profound range may be pacing the hallways of a residence touching the light switches. A care provider tries to redirect the individual to another room, unaware that a ritual is being interrupted. This leads to increased anxiety in the individual who then discharges that anxiety and frustration through an aggressive act.

Aggression and personality disorders. Aggression can also be an associated feature of several personality disorders. Incidents of aggressive or violent behavior can occur among individuals who have an antisocial personality disorder or a borderline personality disorder.

Aggression and substance abuse. It can also occur in response to substance use issues. The possibility of illegal substance use should not be overlooked among individuals who are non-verbal and have an intellectual disability. Unfortunately, there have been situations in which non-verbal individuals, whose cognitive functioning abilities were in the profound and severe ranges, were given drugs by individuals tasked to provide for their care.

Impulse control disorders and aggression. Aggression is a central feature of the diagnosis of Intermittent Explosive Disorder which is an Impulse Control Disorder. This diagnosis is too often given to individuals with an intellectual disability. Impulsive aggression may have many different causes, and this diagnosis is not meant to be given if the aggression can be better accounted for by another mental disorder. It is usually a diagnosis of exclusion or last resort.

2. **Aggression and Medical Disorders.** Aggression can be the result of a medical illness. For example, it can occur in response to the following neurological conditions: a partial complex seizure, stroke, brain abscess, dementia, or a focal frontal lesion (First and Tasman, 2004). Other medical conditions may cause or contribute to aggressive behaviors such as hypoglycemia. Physical discomfort may contribute to aggressive behavior and can occur in response to chronic pain conditions such as arthritis. Aggression may also be the result of

medication side effects and interactions such as medication induced akathisia, disinhibition from sedative/hypnotics, antidepressant use (initial phase), or the side effect of steroid use used to treat an inflammatory condition.

3. **Aggression as a Learned Behavior.** Aggression may not be indicative of a psychiatric disorder. It may be an impulsive response to a stressful situation in the individual's life. Therefore, it is important to assess whether or not the aggression is a sign of an underlying psychiatric issue or simply a response to an abnormal stressful condition. Many individuals with an intellectual disability live under less than optimal situations. They may have less autonomy than others around them. They see others experiencing a variety of privileges and freedoms that they wish they could have. This can lead to frustration and anger. They may have difficulty expressing those feelings and dissatisfactions appropriately. Consequently, aggressive acts may serve as their way of communicating frustrations. Aggression may also be a purposeful behavior that has been reinforced and may occur in order to avoid a task, obtain attention, seek retaliation, obtain a desired object, or intimidate others.

Diagnostic Considerations

In addressing aggression, two errors can occur. The first is the failure to identify an underlying psychiatric condition which may be causing the behavior. This becomes a more difficult task as the severity of the individual's cognitive impairment increases. The second error is in making the wrong diagnosis. These errors can occur as a result of several factors including diagnostic overshadowing (when the behavior is attributed to the developmental disorder itself rather than to a psychiatric condition). In the diagnostic assessment of aggression, it is important to identify any co-occurring symptoms which may help identify a psychiatric disorder. Clinicians may miss the psychiatric diagnosis, or make an incorrect diagnosis, because they focus on the problems associated with the aggression. For example, an individual with autism, who is depressed, may exhibit aggressive behavior in response to the depression. However, the aggression becomes the sole focus of the treatment, thus, missing the fact that the primary condition may be depression.

The diagnosis may also be wrong due factors such as stress. For example, according to Sovner and Hurley (1986), "First, under stress, there is a greater likelihood for individuals with autism to decompensate acutely, a process that has been labeled as Cognitive

Disintegration. These anxiety-based decompensations are sometimes misdiagnosed as psychosis. Yet, this decompensation is likely due to the fact that the individual has limited resources for coping and therefore regressions, and his/her behavior may appear as bizarre" (Homatidis, 2005, p. 56).

Assessment and Treatment of Aggression

Identifying the correct causes of aggression is critical to providing effective treatment. However, determining the exact cause can be a time-consuming process. This can be particularly challenging in light of the need to quickly respond to the behavior and ensure everyone's safety. Further complicating the process is the fact that some behaviors can have multiple causes. Consequently, they may not be occurring in response to just one factor but the combination of several factors. In addition, what may have been the initial cause of the aggression may no longer be the factor that is maintaining the behavior. For example, an individual may have become aggressive because he was in pain and a care provider asked him to move. He may have hit the person in response to being in pain. If the care provider retreated because of the aggression, the individual may have learned that his aggression may provide him with a means of getting people to leave him alone and not make demands on him. Since time to do a comprehensive assessment of the aggression may not always be available due to the potential dangerousness of the behavior, the following questions may assist in expediting the assessment process:

1. Determine if the aggression is a new behavior or a long standing behavior that has just increased.

Is this behavior new? If the presentation is acute, a medical cause should be considered and ruled out. It is not unusual for a simple medical issue such as a migraine headache or a sinus infection to contribute to aggression in individuals with an intellectual disability. If the aggression is chronic, obtain information regarding its history. When did it begin? What were the circumstances in the past which triggered it? If possible, obtain information about how the aggression was addressed. This may provide insight into possible learned elements of the behavior and the contingencies which may have helped sustain it. If it has been chronic, but it has increased recently in severity, explore the possibility of a stress related reaction. Examine current sources of stress for the individual so that stressors may be addressed and alleviated.

Stress related reactions can also produce sudden or quick changes in behavior.

2. Look for any changes in medications including titration schedules (i.e., increases or decreases in medications) or the introduction of a new medication.

Changes in behavior can occur as a result of medication titration schedules or in response to the abrupt withdrawal of certain medications. Medication changes have the potential for de-stabilizing behaviors as well as improving behaviors.

3. Obtain information regarding any current psychiatric diagnoses to determine if aggression is a related feature of that disorder.

For example, if the individual has been diagnosed with Borderline Personality Disorder there may be difficulties regulating emotions and emotional instability.

4. Consider medical causes.

Obtain an update on the individual's medical status and obtain information regarding any recent changes in any health related areas (e.g., eating, elimination patterns, seizure activity). A medical systems review can help identify clues to any underlying medical causes.

5. Assess for any changes in the individual's life.

Has anything recently changed in the person's life? This can include changes in living arrangements or in the individual's support system, such as a recent death or other loss.

Have there been changes in the person's daily routine, etc.?

6. Conduct a brief functional analysis.

There may not be time to do a complete functional analyses but an abbreviated form which answers the following questions may be helpful:

- **Who** –Who does the aggression occur with? Who does it not occur with?
- **What** – What are the situations in which the aggression occurs? External antecedents could include numerous aspects of the environment such as sounds, activities, etc.
- **Where** – Where does it occur and where doesn't it occur?
- **When** – Note the time of day and what is usually occurring during that time?

A fast and quick response to the aggression is often needed, since aggression may escalate to the point that the individual poses an imminent threat to others. According to Ruth Ryan (1996), even at this point in time when people are usually panicked, some basic and careful observations, including the following, may provide some indication of the type of emergency treatment that is needed:

- Vital signs – temperature, blood pressure, and pulse rate
- Mood state – manic, depressed, panicked, rageful
- Thought process – confused, alert, hallucinating, dissociated (such as in a flashback)
- Physical movements – purposeful, perseverative, flailing/uncontrolled, clumsy

If the individual is actively hallucinating, an administration of an antipsychotic medication may be useful as an emergency intervention. If the person appears to be panicked, treatment with an anti-anxiety medication may help in the short term. However, the long-term option of conducting a comprehensive assessment should still be pursued.

Psychiatric Hospitalization and Aggression

A psychiatric hospitalization is sometimes sought for an individual whose aggression has become so frequent or severe that it poses a danger to the community. It is common for aggression to decrease or even stop occurring within a hospital setting. This can lead to a premature discharge from the hospital and a return of the behavior after leaving the hospital resulting in a pattern of recurrent admissions. There are several factors which can account for the absence of the behavior upon admission to the psychiatric facility:

1. The triggers for the aggression may be absent in the environment of the hospital. Upon the individual's discharge and return to the residence, the person may again experience the same triggers. Consequently, the behavior returns.
2. Upon admission, there is a change in the person's social contacts. If the aggression was the result of conflict with a particular care provider or family member, the person may not have contact with that person during the hospital stay. However, upon discharge from the hospital the individual returns to the same situation without having resolved the issue.

3. While in the hospital, the individual is sometimes placed on close observation or even a 1:1 level of supervision. This can be helpful in intervening early so that the individual's behavior does not escalate.
4. Behavior often changes in response to an environmental change (e.g., leaving the home and going to the hospital). However, such changes are usually short-lived.
5. In response to the dangerous behavior which resulted in the hospitalization, the individual may receive an emergency administration of psychotropics. This can result in a level of sedation and a reduction in physical responsiveness.
6. If the aggressive behavior warrants the use of restrictive interventions in the hospital, such as mechanical restraints or physical containment by the staff, these interventions can serve as deterrents to the behavior.

Appendix B

Staff Training

Appendix B includes some general trainings that were offered to an inpatient psychiatric facility that was beginning to work with individuals with dual diagnoses. These trainings were developed for direct care workers who had very little experience working with people with an intellectual disability. Their training was in the mental health field and working with people with psychiatric disorders. The trainings in this section are offered as initial guidelines in understanding the complicating factors of working with people with dual diagnoses. They were included to provide an outline for others being introduced to this field. That said, some of the information may be repeated. Each section was developed as a separate training; therefore, some information is relevant for more than one topic area.

Communication Strategies

Individuals struggling with mental illness often have difficulty concentrating and attending to discussions, particularly when in crisis. If the person has an intellectual disability, it can be even more difficult. When interacting with individuals who have cognitive impairments, it is helpful to modify your language. Here are some guidelines that may be helpful.

1. Keep your language simple and concrete. Point, gesture, model if needed, to assist in making your point. Keep it clear. Reduce your words. Complex instructions, expectations, and questions can be confusing and increase the person's stress level.

2. Explain what you are doing even if you think the person does not understand.

3. Understand that there is a difference between expressive and receptive language. Receptive language refers to the ability to understand language, and expressive language refers to the ability to verbally communicate. Sometimes an individual's expressive language exceeds his or her receptive language which may give the appearance that the person understands more than he or she does. At other times the person understands more than he or she is able to verbally express.

4. Be sensitive to the impact that psychotropic medications can have on a person's ability to process information. Side effects can cause fatigue, lower ability to concentrate, and impact short-term memory. All of these factors can impact a person's ability to maintain a conversation and remember what was said.

5. Avoid multi-step instructions. If too many instructions are strung together, the person may not be able to remember them. Consequently, the person's behavior may be more likely to be viewed as restrictive.

6. Do not talk to the person in a childish manner. Be respectful and adult-like in your communications. They are individuals who are delayed cognitively, but they also have years of life experience.

Common Complaints Expressed by Caregivers

The following are common complaints voiced by residential staff or other care providers when interacting and communicating with individuals with an intellectual disability:

1. *"I have to keep repeating myself."*
   Individuals may perseverate and ask the same questions. There may be one of several things causing this:
   a. The person may be in need of some attention and not know how to effectively initiate or engage in a conversation.
   b. The person may have processing deficits or attentional deficits which impact his or her ability to remember information.
   c. This may be a reflection of an underlying psychiatric condition. Repeated questioning and the need for reassurance can be a symptom of Obsessive Compulsive Disorder or another anxiety disorder such as Generalized Anxiety Disorder. With a Generalized Anxiety Disorder, the individual may be ruminating about issues that are worrisome. Consequently, talking about the sources of the ruminations may be calming for the person.
   d. The individual may be very anxious in anticipation of an event, and this may be a way of dealing with the excitement.
   e. The person may be bored, and this is a way of reducing the boredom

2. "I already told him the answer to his question, *and he repeats it to another staff. He goes from staff to staff with the same question.*"
   This may be the individual's attempt to get a need met, and he or she may not know any other way to obtain the desired goal. By asking several people, the person may hope to eventually obtain the desired answer or action by "wearing people down."

3. "Why am I not seeing any change on a day-to-day basis?"
   Behavior change requires rehearsal of the new skills to be acquired. Insight is also not enough to change behavior. It requires practice of the new skills. In addition, the new behavior should have a "payoff" that is either equal to or larger than the value of the old behavior.

4. "They are so needy."
   Individuals with an intellectual disability often have limited social support networks. Consequently, they may rely on the staff as a significant source of social support.

5. "They are childlike."

The individual may communicate in a childlike way and have some skill deficits in certain areas of development, but it is a mistake to assume the person is childlike. Adults with developmental disorders have the same number of years of life experience as a typically developed adult of the same age.

How to Provide Effective Instructions

When providing instructions to an individual with an intellectual disability, the following basic strategies can be helpful:

- Give choices whenever possible.
- Be specific.
- Keep it simple.
- Check for follow-through and understanding of the instruction.
- If possible, provide a warning around transitions.
  For example, "In ten minutes we will be leaving to go shopping."

Effective Communication Strategies

There are certain communication techniques which can be very helpful in de-escalating situations. These include:

1. **Active listening.**
   This involves reflecting back to the person what you have heard him or her say.
2. **Empathetic responses.**
   There is a difference between sympathy and empathy. Giving a sympathetic response is a response reflecting your feelings. Empathy is the ability to understand another person's feelings and to understand how the person views a situation.
3. **Maintain a non-judgmental attitude.**
   This conveys an attitude that you accept the person and you are not critical. This does not mean that you are necessarily accepting the behavior, just understanding it is important to the person. It is important to maintain a calm, matter-of-fact, and neutral voice. Aggression leads to aggression, i.e., if care providers are verbally aggressive or hostile, it is more likely that the person will react in kind.
4. **Avoid power struggles.**
   It is important in interacting with the people that you work with that you do not get into arguments with them. Avoid being confrontational and avoid arguing with them.

5. **Watch your posture and body language.**
   Avoid any physical stance or posture that can be viewed as challenging.
6. **Validate how they are feeling.**
   You can validate the person's feelings without agreeing with the person.
7. **Put the choices back to the person.**
   If someone's behavior is escalating you can say, "You have a decision to make. You can hit someone or you can…" Put it back on the person and remind the person of the more productive and effective choices that can be made.

Safety Tips in Dealing with Potentially Aggressive Individuals

This training was written for direct support staff who work with aggressive individuals. This may include personnel from hospital or institutional settings or highly supervised residential placements. Provided is a list of things to always be aware of when entering a situation with potential risk:

1. Be aware of who is around you. Have some idea of where your fellow co-workers are in case you need their assistance.

2. Be aware of objects in the environment that can be used as weapons and remove them. The environment should always be monitored to ensure such objects are not readily accessible to any of the individuals should they become agitated. This should also extend to an awareness of any items on your person that can be used as a weapon.

3. Get to know the individuals so you are familiar with the triggers or the antecedents which tend to result in the behavior occurring. Respond as proactively as possible.

4. Monitor the environment for noise level and level of activity. If the television is loud and radios are loud, the environment can be overstimulating, and this can trigger escalating behavioral issues.

5. Watch your own position relative to the person. When interacting with a potentially aggressive person you want to have a door or open space behind you.

6. Watch your tone of voice and your attitude. If you find yourself becoming frustrated or disbelieving of the person, it can show in your communication. If you notice this in yourself, it may be a time to rotate with another staff if possible.

7. Limit setting may be needed.

8. Watch how you dress to ensure your dress does not limit your ability to move quickly or potentially cause injury. For example, if you are a female staff member the heels of your shoes should be low enough to support quick movement. Jewelry can be easily grabbed, and pens can be used to cause injury.

In summary, a staff member who is fully prepared to work with potentially aggressive people is very observant of the environment. That individual has a plan for self-control and is dressed appropriately so as to ensure adequate mobility and personal safety.

Crisis Management and De-Escalation Strategies

Non-Verbal De-Escalation Strategies

It is very important to be skilled at helping to de-escalate an agitated individual. There are both verbal techniques and non-verbal techniques which can be used to de-escalate a situation. Being well prepared to use the non-verbal techniques is very important when working in settings where there are individuals who are prone to exhibit unsafe reactions when agitated.

1. **Monitor your body position and body language.**

   Do not engage in any posturing that can be construed as aggressive or intimidating. For example, don't get in the person's space, point a finger at the person, or give body language cues that signal hostility.

2. **Avoid physically putting yourself in harms way.**

   For example, avoid directly facing an agitated person and putting yourself directly in front of that person. This would make the front of your body fully vulnerable to getting hit. Keep a safe distance of at least 3-4 arm lengths away if not a little more. This will decrease the likelihood of the person grabbing, punching, pulling, or lunging at you. It may be helpful to position yourself at a 45 degree angle to the person. This allows you greater protection of more vulnerable areas. It also allows you a safer retreat if you need it, and it is a non-threatening position to the person. If possible, stand behind a large object. This could include a table, the nursing station, a chair, etc. This provides a possible barrier for you should the person's agitation continue.

3. **Maintain a demeanor of calmness, neutrality, and confidence.**
   You want to present with a non-judgmental demeanor but one that indicates you are also attentive. If the person is feeling out-of-control, he or she needs to know that someone around them is going to take control if needed. This gives the person a sense of security. Monitor your own self-talk. If you are telling yourself, "I'm in trouble. What am I going to do?" this will only lead to anxiety and possibly panic on your part, and it will prevent you from thinking and acting more clearly and effectively. Instead, substitute that thinking for more constructive, positive self-talk, such as "I can handle this. I have options. I can also get assistance."

Verbal De-escalation Strategies

1. **Use a calm tone of voice.**
   Avoid showing any strong emotional reaction to the person.

2. **Use reflective listening.**
   Reflect back the feelings you think you are hearing and seeing. For example, "I know that must have really upset you."

3. **Avoid threatening punishment.**
   You can remind the person of the possible consequences of his or her actions without threatening punishment. For example, you can say "Now remember, you are working toward that weekend pass."

4. **Avoid power struggles.**
   It is important the person feels his or her views are important and valid. Getting into a conversation about who is "right" can cause a power struggle, so avoid those conversations.

5. **Do not ignore escalations of behaviors that could lead to severe behaviors.**
   Intervene as early in the stages of escalation as possible.

6. **Change staffing if necessary.**
   If the individual is very angry at you, it would not be helpful to continue to try and deal with that person. Have another staff take over. Otherwise the person is likely to continue staying agitated in your presence. Also, if you feel you can no longer deal with a person effectively on that shift because of your own emotional reactions, ask another staff to assist or take over. We are only human. Another staff can intervene to redirect the individual to another activity or let him or her vent appropriately.

7. **Affirm that you understand.**
   You do not need to communicate that you agree with the person's perspective. Simply understanding that whatever happened was upsetting for that person can be very validating. Understanding the individual's perspective does not mean you are necessarily agreeing with it.

8. **Change the subject if it appears to agitate the person more to talk about it.**
   Help the individual focus on something else. If he or she keeps ruminating about the issue that caused the anger, the agitation will continue.

9. **Change aspects of the environment.**
    For example, decrease stimulation in the environment in order to produce a more calming and peaceful environment. Simply turning off a T.V. or moving people out of the room can have a calming effect.
10. **Be limit setting by reminding the person of the rules but do so in a firm, fair manner and with a non-emotional tone of voice.**
11. **Remind the individual of the undesirable consequences that can occur if he or she engages in the behavior**

Common mistakes that could increase agitation.

The following interventions have the capability of either increasing the agitation or re-escalating the situation. These are things to be *avoided*:

* Responding with verbal aggressiveness or abruptness
* Ignoring the individual's needs
* Taking away all choices
* Using threats of the loss of privileges

Management Strategies for Working with Challenging Behaviors

1. **Take a more objective approach.**

   Instead of viewing challenging behaviors as annoying, frustrating, etc., view the behaviors as serving a function. They serve a communicative function. The behaviors communicate a need or needs that the individual has. That individual may be trying to get a need met in the only way he or she knows how. View all problem behavior as having meaning, even if that meaning is a reflection of a medical need or a psychiatric condition. For example, the behavior could mean "I'm tired." "I'm lonely." "I'm scared." A single behavior can reflect several needs. It is not uncommon for one of the underlying needs to be a need for attention, tension release, avoidance, escape, or play.

2. **Use challenging moments as "teachable moments."**

   When the person is starting to exhibit some challenging and disruptive behavior, think in terms of how that individual can get his or her need met in a more adaptive way and focus on the replacement behavior. This may be an opportunity to help him or her learn how to get his or her needs met more effectively and learn specific coping and life skills. If a replacement behavior is not identified, either the challenging behavior will continue to be strengthened or another equally inappropriate behavior will be exhibited.

3. **Avoid power struggles.**

   It takes two to make an argument. Sometimes a potential argument can be deflated by using a response such as "I understand." You are not agreeing with the individual, just simply acknowledging that you understand how the person is looking at the situation and feeling about it. Don't get drawn into arguments. Don't threaten punishment as this could serve to escalate behavior. For example, in a hospital setting if a staff says, "If you do that you will lose your pass" it may not produce the same results as, "Remember, you have a pass you worked hard for. I would hate to see you not have that pass because of this behavior." Intervene with a calm demeanor and with clear limit-setting that is done with the presentation of choices and options. For example, "I see you are upset. I know you have worked hard for that pass, and if you hit someone you won't be able to use it. Why don't I help you get space from others so you can feel calmer?"

4. **Provide choices whenever possible**.

   People who have been admitted to a hospital involuntarily are often feeling as though they have no control over their situation, since that is not where they want to be. Sometimes just presenting choices whenever appropriate can help foster cooperation and help the person to feel better. The choice can be a forced choice such as, "Do you want to take a bath after medications are given or before?" Avoid giving ultimatums but rather give choices when possible.

5. **Help establish some routine in the day**.

   The routine should include some opportunities for leisure skills and recreational activities. If there is too much unstructured time, this could lead to behavioral challenges.

   One of the kindest things you can give someone is structure. This makes the world more predictable and lessens anxiety.

6. **When setting limits do so in a clear and concise manner**.

   For example, "Katie, you need to step away from the door or you will have to return to the unit." It is easier to be clear if the limit is set with as few words as possible. Also, offer an explanation of the consequence if the behavior continues.

7. **If you want a person to stop a behavior, think in terms of what other behavior you would like to see exhibited**.

8. **Don't take the behavior personally**.

9. **Don't forget the power of praise and positive reinforcement**.

10. **Avoid operating in a reactive mode**.

    Sometimes care providers adopt the attitude of not bothering the person if he or she is not exhibiting any behavior problems. If this is the case, what is the payoff for good behavior? Sometimes this can then lead to negative behavior out of boredom or the need for attention. Episodic, severe behavior may be a reflection of a decay in the program. Providing a great deal of attention after a problem behavior has been exhibited, and then decreasing the attention over the next few days, until it happens again, can lead to future escalations of the behavior.

11. **Help create safety zones for the person**.

    Individuals, particularly those in institutionalized or psychiatric settings, need safe, quiet areas to go.

12. **Intervene early.**

    Intervene early at the first sign of a problem in order to avoid a further escalation. Problem behaviors often occur as part of a behavioral chain or sequence. Interrupting this chain early in the sequence can prevent further escalation. For example, the use of proximity control (relocating the individual) or instructional control (providing verbal prompts) can be helpful.

13. **Understand that transitions can be difficult.**

    Because transitions can be difficult, help prepare the individual for the anticipated changes. Transitions which involve a person moving out of a facility to the community, beginning a new job program, or going to a medical appointment can be difficult. The person may need some extra support in preparing for transitions both on a behavioral and on an emotional level.

14. **Monitor the environment.**

    Ensure that the environment is not too overstimulating. Change the location and time of activities if those factors are contributing to behavioral challenges. Also monitor the environment to ensure that objects which that be tempting are removed. For example, if someone is known to tear down pictures when mad, it may be beneficial to move them or bolt them down.

15. **Facilitate communication.**

    When someone starts to show early signs of agitation, make an effort to determine the problem. Help the person communicate his or her concern in a safe way.

16. **Use the Premack Principle.**

    This has also been referred to as "Grandma's Rule." It refers to using the opportunity to engage in a high probability behavior as a motivator to perform a low probability behavior. For example, "Take your shower first so then you can watch television." This is assuming that the behavior of taking a shower is really a low preference or undesirable behavior and that watching television is a highly preferred activity. This strategy can be very effective in getting someone to perform a behavior they need to do but have little desire to do it. It is best when it is offered before the person expresses dissatisfaction with the request.

17. **Follow through on promises.**

    Do not make promises that you may not be able to keep.

18. **Get to know the person.**
    The more you learn about a person, the better chance you have of dealing with his or her challenging behavior in the most effective way. Learn about the person's history as it pertains to the current behaviors and situation. Learn the triggers, both environmentally and interpersonally, that can lead to problem behaviors. Learn what the person likes and what is motivating to him or her.

19. **Help the person to feel good about himself or herself.**
    Help the person to develop a positive identity and accentuate the positives.

Working with Families

Family Dynamics

The following are some common dynamics that are present in families of individuals with developmental disorders:

- There may be some denial of the extent of their son or daughter's mental illness.
- They may have a lack of understanding with regard to how the mental health issues may be impacting behaviors.
- There may be a history of inappropriate behaviors being rewarded. Due to such factors as guilt, the family may reinforce inappropriate behaviors because they may feel guilty over having placed their son or daughter in a group home or institution. They may also have some guilt if they felt the intellectual disability was caused by genetic factors or a traumatic event. In addition, the stressors experienced by the family may have them resorting to the "path of least resistance." Therefore, the problematic behaviors are rewarded because family members do not have the energy to be consistent and establish consequences. Taking the path of least resistance may also result in a lack of structure in the home which can contribute to the behavioral challenges.
- It is not unusual for families to either be too enmeshed and try to run to the person's rescue or to be distant and non-involved. The non-involvement can be felt by the individual and experienced as a chronic sense of loss and longing, given the fact that often the individual has a limited social support system.
- Family members may sabotage or undermine the person's treatment. For example, a family may bring the person cigarettes when the person is on a program to limit smoking. Families have their ways in which they have tried to control the behaviors. Unfortunately, sometimes that has involved a response that has only served to exacerbate the behaviors and reward maladaptive behaviors. For example, they may have told their daughter they will give her that item she wants if she stops screaming about it.

How to Address Potentially Conflictual Situations with Families

Difficult interactions can be triggered by several factors:

- The family's frustration over a lack of services for their son or daughter

- Discouragement
- Guilt
- Misunderstandings about the course of treatment and services available

How to deal with difficult interactions:

- There is a need for active listening so that the concerns, fears, and frustrations of the family can be heard.
- Be empathetic.
- Be assertive when needed, but not verbally confrontational.
- Try to obtain their involvement and assistance as part of the treatment team.
- Obtain a history of the individual's relationship with their parents and other family members so that any emotional trigger points can be identified.
- Understand that if there is discussion of having a person move from an institutionalized setting to the community this could evoke a range of emotional responses from family members.
- Maintain effective boundaries.

Boundaries Between Professionals and Adults with an Intellectual Disability

When working with people with dual diagnoses it is easy to lose sight of personal boundaries. Care providers spend a lot of time with the people they serve and learn about them on an intimate level. At the same time, they are not peers or family members. Adults with dual diagnoses have more difficulty understanding this relationship than the professional. Therefore, it is the professional's responsibility to maintain the boundary as a coach, model, and teacher.

It is imperative to maintain healthy, professional boundaries when working with people with dual diagnoses. Many difficulties with human relationships can be reduced to difficulties with boundaries. Either boundaries were not well defined or they were enmeshed, or too strict, etc. There are different types of boundaries, including physical, emotional, and financial boundaries. In order to establish healthy boundaries in working with people the following elements are important to consider:

1. You can develop a warm relationship while still being professional.
2. Avoid thinking or behaving as though you are the only person who can deal with that individual. This introduces a host of potential difficulties for that person and the other staff members. It can result in the person encouraging the staff to feel adversarial toward each other. It could also result in a lack of consistency in implementing behavioral strategies.
3. Be sensitive to gender issues. Respect the privacy of the individual. Be prudent and respectful of privacy in supervising an individual's personal care needs. Avoid being alone with a person of the opposite sex.
4. Don't talk about personal issues in front of the people you are assisting.
5. Remember that attachments can develop quicker among individuals with an intellectual disability.
6. Monitor your language and tone of voice. Be respectful in your interactions. Watch your tone of voice. Remember that aggression leads to aggression. This includes not just physical aggression but verbal aggression. When you are setting limits do so with respectful language and a respectful tone. In addition, remember that negative comments about individuals can be harmful to them.

7. There may be a propensity to "baby" the individual because of the intellectual disability. Even though the person may have some cognitive deficits, this individual also has years of life experience that he or she is bringing to the interaction.

8. Be careful and monitor when the individual says things like "I love you" or "Mommy." Correct those situations and politely, tell the person how you want to be addressed. Allowing the person to use such terms speaks to the development of a different type of relationship than a professional one. Individuals may develop romantic feelings toward staff members. Always clarify the staff/client relationship. Report any of these behaviors on the part of the person to the supervisor or case manager and document. This also helps protect you against future false allegations.

9. Be consistent. If you are not consistent, you may set up other staff members or care providers for conflict with the individual.

10. Do not lend an individual you are caring for money or buy them gifts. To give an individual money or gifts is extending the relationship beyond the client-staff relationship.

11. Avoid making deals and compromises. This means you should avoid trying to get a person to cooperate with a request by giving them a promise of special privileges.

Maintaining Professional Boundaries

If you are a staff member or other professional working with an individaul, it is very important to maintain professional boundaries for a variety of reasons. If the individual has had significant problems in his or her relationships with others, maintaining good boundaries can provide the individual with corrective experiences. It is also important for teaching social skills. In addition, providing consistency in interpersonal interactions is critical for the implementation of behavioral intervention plans. Without this consistency, the individual may receive confusing messages from others, and this can undermine a team approach and encourage staff splitting.

Friendship versus a professional relationship. The relationship between the individual and a staff member must center around the purpose of placement and active treatment. It should never involve a relationship based on friendship. Individuals may want more contact and ask for contact that is outside of the professional relationship. For example, they may ask to meet the staff member's children or go to a staff member's home, etc. Always maintain a professional relationship. Individuals with an intellectual disability may develop relationships quicker and become very reliant on staff. This is due to several factors:

1. They may have limited social support network. Friendships have not been fostered, and individuals may not have had the social opportunities to develop and maintain friendships.

2. There may be a lack of social skills training. Interpersonal difficulties can also be the result of long standing unhealthy patterns of relating to people. For example, it is not uncommon for individuals with a diagnosis of Borderline Personality Disorder to engage in inappropriate social behavior with others as a way to interact or connect, and in doing so they may cross personal or physical boundaries.

3. There may be a history of losses including not having contact with their family of origin.

4. People have felt sorry for them based on their diagnosis of intellectual disability and engender dependency rather than autonomy. They begin to rely heavily on others because they don't feel competent.

5. Staff may work intensely with individuals during treatment, and this can lead to feelings of attachment to the staff.

Introductory Guidelines for Some Common Psychiatric Disorders

These guidelines were developed to assist support staff in working with people with dual diagnoses. They were not meant to replace a comprehensive plan. In fact, the guidelines are brief. Instead, they were developed as a starting point and to provide things to consider when working with individuals who struggle with these disorders.

Interventions for Supporting Someone with Psychosis

The important thing to remember when working with persons who are experiencing psychotic symptoms, whether they are hallucinations or delusions, is to provide a safe, supportive environment as much as possible. In addition, their beliefs are strong and they are likely to be frightened of, angry at, or dismiss anyone who challenges those beliefs. If you argue with them about their delusions, they may become distrustful. If you challenge their delusions, you are challenging their grasp on reality. If they are frightened by the delusions, just acknowledge the emotion and assist them in trying to feel safe. For example, if they have a paranoid delusion that the people in the room are talking about them and it is frightening them, encourage them to go to another area so they can feel safe. Also, try and redirect the conversation to more reality based topics.

1. Do not challenge or support their delusions. Do not agree or disagree.
2. Avoid joking about any of their delusions.
3. Reduce environmental stimuli.
4. Add structure. External structure can be helpful because they are lacking the internal structure. This structure should be flexible to allow for change when the person is feeling uncomfortable.
5. Talk with them in a calm, direct manner.
6. Reduce stress.

Interventions for Individuals with Borderline and Histrionic Personality Disorders

The key when working with individuals with Borderline or Histrionic Personality Disorders is to monitor your relationship with the person you are working with. The core of these personality disorders is relational and how others respond to them. These guidelines will focus on how the maintain boundaries and structured communication with people with these disorders.

1. **BOUNDARIES, BOUNDARIES, BOUNDARIES**

Always maintain professional, physical, and personal boundaries. You can be warm, polite, and friendly while maintaining good boundaries.

   a. Offer handshakes and high-fives instead of hugs.
   b. Share limited information about your personal life.
   c. Avoid nicknames unless it is house-wide.
   d. Socialize in public parts of the residence.

2. **Be very consistent among staff.**

Staff need to support each other. Anytime the person brings a staff-related issue to you, make sure to always check with the staff before responding.

3. **Be consistent with what you say.**

Often the person will bring the same issue to you over and over again. Choose a simple four to five word response and politely give the same response over and over. Part of what the person is looking for is the chance that you will change your mind or a way to make you upset and get a reaction. In addition, the person may also be testing you for predictability. Predictability creates safety, and this may be a way for the person to develop trust.

4. **Stay problem-solving focused.**

When communicating about high stress topics, it is a good rule of thumb to talk about what the person thinks and not how he or she feels. Focus on the outcome the person is seeking and what needs to happen to get that outcome. Don't challenge the persons ideas, just walk him or her through the process. For example, "You want to move out and want to tell the service coordinator you are leaving this week. Okay, I can help you call her. What I am thinking is that if you call her and want to move soon, your choices might be limited. What do you think about calling her and asking her what the process would be to find a home more of your choice?"

5. **Validate the person.**

In high risk or agitated situations, it can be helpful to simply validate the person's feelings. You can validate the person's feelings without agreeing with what the person is saying. For example:

"I can tell that made you really mad."

"I can see how sad you are.

"You are really upset."

6. **Tag team**.

   If one staff person is the target of anger or an irrational attack, have someone else work with that individual. That person can validate the individual's feelings without getting involved in the conflict. For example:

   "I am not sure what they meant, but I can see you are mad."

   "We will figure that out later. Right now I can see how upset you are and I want to help you feel better."

7. **Provide low energy reactions**.

   Use a matter-of-fact tone of voice and avoid conflicts about irrational issues.

8. **Structure is important.**

   Individuals with borderline characteristics do better with structure in their environment. This provides consistency which often translates to safety.

9. **Confrontation is not helpful.**

   The person often does not understand confrontation because of boundary problems. Being directive also does not work because it can be perceived as controlling.

10. **Anything that involves catharsis is not helpful.**

    When a person with borderline or histrionic characteristics is encouraged to "let it all out", it tends to lead to regression and losing control of the emotion. This can feel scary and uncomfortable for the person. It is also often difficult for the person to pull it back together safely.

11. **Let them experience the natural consequences of their behaviors.**

    This can be an important lesson in how behavior impacts others. People with these personality disorders tend to focus on their internal reactions and don't attend to how their behavior is impacting those around them. In addition, behavioral reactions can be impulsive without thought of long-term consequences. Experiencing natural consequences communicates the impact of their behavioral reaction.

12. **Be aware of your own reaction.**

    This can be a challenging group of people to work with. It can lead to frustration and low patience. This often stems from the care provider feeling the person is being manipulative and self-focused. It is important to be honest with yourself if you are getting frustrated because it can show in your interactions. This group tends to be hypersensitive to the reactions of others. If you feel frustrated, it may be time to alternate care with someone else for a brief time.

13. **Be a "feelings coach."**

   Individuals with these diagnoses tend to act on their emotions. They feel them and then without thinking about the consequences of their behavior, they act on them. It is important to teach them appropriate ways to communicate how they are feeling. For example, "I can see you are mad at your boyfriend. When you yell and scream it is distracting, and I can't hear what you are saying about him. Let's take some deep breaths and talk quieter so I can listen."

Interventions for Individuals with Obsessive-Compulsive Disorder

The key when working with someone who has Obsessive-Compulsive Disorder is to assess the degree to which the compulsive behavior is a risk to harm the person or someone else or interfere with the person's daily functioning. The direct intervention will differ depending on the intensity and need to change it for safety.

1. **Assess whether the behavior is safe or unsafe.**

   If the behavior is safe you may not have to help the person change it. If the behavior is safe, but interferes with daily functioning, the intervention may not be as intense. For example, if the person has an ordering compulsion and needs to organize the chairs around a table, it may not need to be changed. If the person has a checking compulsion and needs to check locks and drawers repetitively before leaving the house, it may interfere with the ability to get somewhere on time or even leave the house. This would need to be addressed, but is not an imminent risk. If the person has a skin picking compulsion, it could lead to serious injury. This would need to be addressed intensely and quickly.

2. **Offer alternatives.**
   a. You can simply ask the person to stop.
   b. Offer something else to do in place of the behavior.
   c. Help the person become involved in another activity.
   d. Offer a preferred activity.
   e. Offer an incongruent activity, something that does not allow the person to engage in the compulsive behavior while doing it. For example, if the person picks his or her skin, hand massages or making sculptures out of clay might help.

3. **Change the environment.**
   a. If you are out, go somewhere else.

b. If you are at home, go for a walk or go outside.

c. Change the people who are around the individual.

d. Remove the tempting item.

4. **Prepare for the reaction if a ritual or compulsive behavior is interrupted.**

You are likely to see a lot of agitation and frustration if it is stopped. Prepare for the chance that the person will become aggressive or unsafe in response to interrupting or preventing the ritualistic or compulsive behavior from occurring. Decide if the negative reaction is worth stopping the behavior at that time.

5. **Obtain a psychiatric consultation for medication.**

If the OCD symptoms are of moderate to severe intensity, medication may be effective.

6. **Consider a Sensory Integration Disorder as a contributing factor.**

If a person is experiencing sensory input in a manner that is significantly more or less than typical, it can result in a sensory integration disorder. A person may react to the sensory input with compulsive behavior. An occupational therapy consultation is important to rule-out the possibility. If a sensory integration disorder exists, there are several interventions that can be very effective.

Interventions for Posttraumatic Stress Disorder

The key when working with a person who is suffering with PTSD is to provide a safe environment that is void of any stimuli that reminds the person of the traumatic event. For this reason it is helpful to identify what the traumatic event was and the circumstances surrounding the event if possible.

1. Obtain a medical evaluation to ensure there are not underlying medical conditions which can be contributing to the psychiatric symptoms. For example, symptoms of panic can be the result of PTSD. They can also be the result of various medical conditions.

2. Obtain a psychiatric consultation to determine if medications may be helpful.

3. Obtain as much information as possible about the circumstances of the abuse. Conduct an ongoing trigger analysis (i.e., a functional analysis of the triggers for the flashbacks). This can provide essential information about what type of setting would feel safest for the person. In addition,

it can provide information about which staff members the person may be most comfortable with (i.e., male or female, soft-spoken or animated, etc.).

4. Identify potential triggering events and help create a safe environment. Change aspects of the environment in order to avoid any trauma triggers. In addition, it can help identify whether the approach of the care providers will impact the person's feeling of safety. For example, awareness of voice tone and body cues are typically important when working with someone with PTSD.

5. Provide training for staff and family. Front line staff are unfortunately some of the last ones to learn about PTSD and the first ones to be assaulted when they inadvertently trigger a traumatic memory for the individual. Knowledge about the trauma can be helpful in reducing the chance the person will re-experience the trauma and in reducing the risk of inadvertently harming a caretaker..

6. Avoid coercive strategies or environments that are too controlling. It is important to allow choice and the opportunity to avoid stressful situations when possible.

7. The use of seclusion, heavy sedation, or any punitive interventions are contraindicated. This can cause the person to feel threatened and can re-traumatize the person.

8. Do not require the person to have contact with any abusers. This undermines their recovery and disrupts the individual's ability to trust in the system.

9. If the individual is experiencing flashbacks, reassurance and reorientation are the primary emphasis. It is important to help "ground" the person in the here-and-now.

10. Refer the person for individual therapy if appropriate based on the cognitive functioning of that person.

11. A safe and healing environment is essential when working with this population. Therefore, considering the peer group living in the home with the person is important. For example, if the person is easily frightened by loud voices or yelling, it will be important he or she is not living with someone who yells or is aggressive.

Appendix C

Group Training and Activities

Activities for use in:
- Group Therapy
- Individual Therapy
- Independent Living Skills Group
- Individual Coaching
- Group Home
- Individual Plan
- Day Program

This section includes activities and worksheets that can be included in a group therapy or group skills curriculum. They could also very easily be adapted when working with people individually in a variety of settings. Here is a list of the topics included in this section.

Topic: **SOCIAL SKILLS**
Sessions: 1. Relaxation Skills
            2. Initiating Conversations
            3. Expressing Feelings
            4. Dealing with Accusation

Topic: **PERSONAL BOUNDARIES**
Sessions: 1. Personal Space
            2. Boundaries and Touch
            3. Boundaries and Conversation

Topic: **LEISURE SKILLS**

Sessions: 1. Leisure Activities and Times to Enjoy Them

Topic: **MONEY MANAGEMENT**

Sessions: 1. Collecting and Monitoring Money

2. Spending and Monitoring Money

Topic: **SELF-CARE**

Sessions: 1. Hygiene-appearance

2. Hygiene-body odor (can be combined with session 1)

3. Privacy

4. Medication

Topic: **WORK READINESS**

Sessions: 1. Developing Work Readiness Skills

2. Job Match

3. Responsible Workplace Behavior

SOCIAL SKILLS

Sessions: 1.   Relaxation Skills
            2.   Initiating Conversations
            3.   Expressing Feelings
            4.   Dealing with an Accusation

GOAL: To learn the skills to interact in a socially appropriate manner in various settings.

Relaxation Skills

Goal: To develop the skills necessary to remain calm when feeling upset.

Objective: To be able to identify high energy feelings and learn relaxation skills to cope with them safely.

Group Discussion:

I. People are more likely to act without thinking and do something they shouldn't when they have *high energy feelings*. High energy feelings are when your body feels a lot of energy that is hard to control. People can have different experiences of high energy feelings. They can feel different for each of us. What makes us feel this way can also be different for each of us.
   a. tingly feeling
   b. nauseous stomach
   c. tight muscles
   d. hard to sit still
   e. tapping foot or fingers quickly
   f. talking loud and fast
   e. *"Any others?"*

II. What are some *high energy feelings*?
   a. angry
   b. excited
   c. nervous
   d. *"Yes, sad or depressed can be a high energy feeling for some people."*

III. What can you do to decrease the energy so you can deal with it better and safer?

*"***TOP THREE***"*

We are going to call the things that you like the best to calm your energy when you are feeling this way your "Top Three"

I am going to give you some ideas and maybe you will have more to teach me.

1. ***Buddha Belly***
   Sit in relaxed position with arms and legs uncrossed
   Take a deep breath into your belly (not you chest)
   Let your belly (diaphragm) fill with air like you just ate a big meal
   As you breathe in silently count to five in a calm way

Let your breath out and count to five in a calm way
Let's practice. I will count for you.

2. **PMR – Progressive Muscle Relaxation**
   Sit in a relaxed position with arms and legs uncrossed
   Squeeze fists together tight and slowly count to five
   release and slowly count to five
   Squeeze stomach tight and slowly count to five release
   and slowly count to five
   Squeeze legs tight and slowly count to five release and
   slowly count to five
   Repeat for any other body parts that are tense

3. **Rocket**
   Press hands together in a praying pose in front of you
   (like a rocket)
   Push hands together and slowly count to five as you
   breathe in slowly
   Relax the squeeze and calmly raise your hands
   (like a rocket taking off) and bring them down to your
   side in half circles away from your body while breathing
   out to a slow five count. Repeat as necessary.

IV.   Are there other things that you find relaxing?
   a.   music (playing or listening)
   b.   doing puzzles
   c.   taking a walk
   d.   exercise (weights, dance, etc.)
   e.   watching T.V.
   f.   writing

Group Activity:

   Help the residents practice and learn the "TOP THREE." Also help them develop at least two or three other activities they find relaxing. Make a picture or collage of the relaxing activities of their choice so they can learn that when someone asks them if they want help with their "TOP THREE" it will be familiar to them. The person may substitute an alternate activity for their "TOP THREE" if one of the relaxation exercises is not comfortable for them or is difficult to do.

   NOTE: People often make up their own relaxation movements. These are all great and should be encouraged. Support the person by having him or her teach you the movement.

Initiating Conversations

Goal:　　　　To develop the skills to initiate conversations and promote socialization.

Objective:　To be able to initiate a conversation at the appropriate time and with pro-social skills.

Group Discussion:

I.　What are some times you might want to start a conversation with someone?
   - a. staff person at your home
   - b. new person at the hospital
   - c. receptionist
   - d. co-worker
   - e. boss
   - f. family member
   - g. peer
   - h. *"Any others?"*

II.　What do you need to remember when approaching someone?
   - a. Remember, it is always important to look pleasant to get the best response.
     - 1. smile
     - 2. relaxed body posture
     - 3. eye contact
   - b. Notice whether they are doing something or talking to someone.
   - c. Are you interrupting something or are they waiting and ready to be approached?

III.　What do you do when you are ready to start talking to the person?
   - a. Look at the person with a smile.
   - b. Use a pleasant tone of voice.
   - c. Ask a question to start the conversation.
   - d. Don't interrupt them when they are talking.

IV.　Conversation Starters: A question or comment to begin a conversation.

What are some ways that you might want to start a conversation?
   - a. "Hi, my name is... ."
   - b. "How long have you worked (lived) here?"
   - c. "What is your name?"
   - d. "Do you like working here?"

    e. "Do you like living here?"

V. Conversation Connectors: Follow up the person's answer with a related question. When the person answers you, it is good that ask them something about what they said.

    a. "What other type of jobs have you had?"

    b. "What do you like to do with your free time?"

    c. "Do you know... (another co-worker or resident)?"

    d. "Where else have you lived?"

Group Activity:

Model how to initiate a conversation. Show examples of the body language of someone who may want to be approached and someone who may not want to be approached. Then use a "conversation starter" and "conversation connector." Then have the residents practice initiating conversations.

Expressing Feelings

Goal: To develop the skills necessary to communicate feelings in a proactive and effective manner.

Objective: To be able to monitor behavior and communicate feelings in a safe way.

Group Discussion:

I.   What feelings may you want to express?
- a. frustration
- b. anger
- c. sadness
- d. happiness

II. There are three things to remember when you want the person to pay attention to what you are saying:

GOOD VOICE

GOOD FACE

GOOD BODY

III. GOOD VOICE means:
- a. quiet tone
- b. no threats
- c. talk slowly

IV. GOOD FACE means:
- a. relaxed face
- b. don't scrunch up your face
- c. good eye contact

V. GOOD BODY means:
- a. relaxed posture
- b. slow movements
- c. hands down to your side and unclenched
- d. give good personal space (at least two arm lengths, if you can touch them you are too close)

VI. You may need some time to help your body get this way before approaching someone to talk to them about how you are feeling. Things you can do are:
- a. take deep breaths
- b. listen to music
- c. take a walk
- d. practice your "TOP THREE"

Group Activity:

Have group members stand up and see what the body postures look like. Point out how they feel when someone approaches them with a relaxed open posture versus an angry body posture.

      a. hold their body tense, clench their fist, scrunch their face, talk loud

      b. take deep breaths to relax the body (in for a count of 5 and out for 5)

      c. tense body parts for a count of 5 and relax for a count of 5 (arms, legs, stomach, face)

      d. hold their body relaxed, arms relaxed, calm facial expression, quiet voice

      e. repeat two or three times

Dealing with an Accusation

Goal: To develop the skills necessary to cope with dealing with an accusation that makes them hurt or angry.

Objective: To be able to learn the skills to identify hurt and angry feelings and respond when they feel they are treated unfairly.

Group Discussion:

I. When a person says something negative about you that is not true it can make you feel:

  a. angry
  b. sad
  c. confused
  d. "Any others?"

II. Here are some guidelines on how to respond in a way that you can get your feelings heard and not get you in trouble.

  a. Practice your "TOP THREE"
   1. Buddha Belly – deep breathing
   2. PMR – progressive muscle relaxation
   3. Rocket – diaphragm opening
   4. Others you find helpful
  b. Remain calm
  c. Do not say anything right away
  d. It is okay to walk away if you are not remaining calm

III. To address the person and share your feelings:

  a Look at the person with a calm facial expression.
  b. Remain calm and be aware of your feelings and behavior.
   1. Are you feeling more angry?
   2. Does your body look threatening?
   3. Are you feeling tense?
   4. Is your face still calm?
  c. Listen completely to what the other person is saying
   1. Don't interrupt
   2. Give good eye contact
  d. Acknowledge what the person is saying
   1. I understand you felt..."
   2. "When I did that you thought..."
   3. Ask if this is the appropriate time to respond.

Say, "May I respond to what you are saying?"

4. If the person says "Yes", then respond truthfully about what you thought happened.

5. Remember, GOOD VOICE, GOOD FACE, GOOD BODY

6. Stay calm

7. If the person says "No," delay your disagreement to a later time and continue to listen.

IV. If the other person is not polite you can:

    a. Continue to listen calmly.

    b. Say, "I am not going to listen to you yell at me."

    c. Say, "Let's get a staff person to help us with this."

    d. Walk away calmly and ask for help.

Group Activity:

Role-play scenarios and situations. If the group members are uncomfortable participating in this exercise, the group leaders can provide appropriate and inappropriate scenarios on the part of each person in the disagreement.

PERSONAL BOUNDARIES

Sessions: 1. Personal Space
               2. Boundaries and Touch
               3. Boundaries and Conversation

GOAL: The goal for this module is to assist residents in
               developing and maintaining appropriate boundaries
               to protect and respect themselves and others when it
               comes to personal contact with others.

Personal Space

Goal: To protect and respect the personal space of themselves and others.

Objective: To identify and respect the distance they should stand from others, including friends, strangers, and family.

Group Discussion:

I.   What is personal space?
  a. The distance that your body is from another person's body when:
    1. sitting
    2. talking
    3. standing in line or in a group
  b. How much space do you want when:
    1. sitting
    2. talking
    3. standing in line or in a group
  c. The "Rule of Thumb" when being respectful of someone's personal space is to stand at least one arm's distance from the person.
      (It is really helpful to provide a visual cue rather than giving an abstract statement such as "give me space." The arm's distance rule can be communicated non-verbally by holding out your arm and verbally by saying "I need arm's distance.")

II. Why is personal space important?
  a. How do you feel when someone is standing too close?
  b. How would someone else feel when you are standing too close?

III. How does the amount of personal space differ depending on the person?
  a. Who do you allow to cross your personal boundary (friends, family, strangers, significant others)?
  b. Who don't you allow to cross your personal boundary (friends, family, strangers, significant others)?

Activity: Hula Hoops

Ask for one or two volunteers and offer them each a hula hoop. Stand in the hula hoop and rest it comfortably on your back. Then demonstrate that the hula hoop is approximately one arm's distance away. Walk up to your volunteers and show them that they are approximately one arm's distance away. Walk around the room slowly with the volunteers and stop when your hula hood touches someone. This activity can be done with all members of the group. Allow them the opportunity to see what a personal circle of space is. This can then be used as a discussion tool when someone is not respecting personal space. You can remind the person of the hula hoop or "arm's distance." Visual cues are very effective learning tools.

Boundaries and Touch

Goal: To protect and respect the bodies of themselves and others.

Objective: To identify and respect behavior and parts of their body that are private, as well as how to maintain boundaries.

Group Discussion:

I. Your body is yours, and you and only you get to decide who touches any part of your body. Everyone is different and no one should push you to do something you are not comfortable with.

II. Define your boundaries as they relate to how comfortable you are being touched.
   a. Are you affectionate and like hugs?
   b. Do you like to have your own space and not be touched?
   c. Do you only like to be touched by people you are close to?
   d. Do you only like to be touched when you are in a talkative and friendly mood?

III. Communicating your boundaries about being touched.
   a. How do you tell people you don't want to be touched?
   b. Are there some people that don't respect your wishes?
   c. What can you do when someone does not respect your wishes?

IV. Other people communicating the boundaries about being touched to you.
   a. Do you tend to stand close up or far away from people when you are talking to them?
   b. Do people need to remind you sometimes that you are standing too close?
   c. What do you do when they remind you?

V. Identify one person you would tell if someone is touching you or has touched you and you don't like it.
   a. Is that person always available to you?
   b. Do you have a way to contact them?
   c. For what purpose would you contact them?

Activity: Privacy Circles

Have group members draw pictures of or put the names of people they would put in each of the circles; people who it is okay to put their arm around or hold their hand, hug and kiss, and not touch at all. This offers the opportunity to discuss friends, strangers, family, significant others, etc. Don't forget to include people they don't want to touch them at all.

PRIVACY CIRCLES

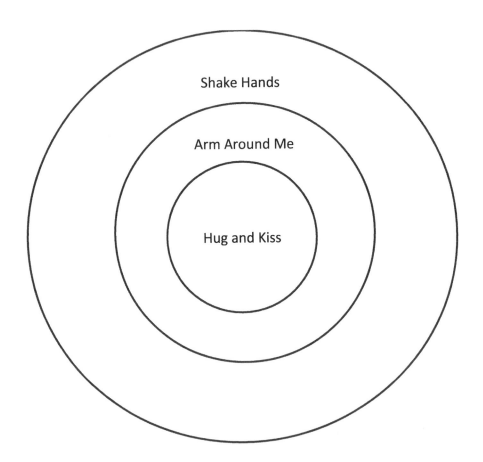

Shake Hands

Arm Around Me

Hug and Kiss

DON'T TOUCH ME!!!

Boundaries and Conversation

Goal: To protect and respect the privacy of themselves and
             others.

Objective: To identify and respect topics of conversation that are
             okay and that are inappropriate to share with others.
             Also, to identify different people with whom to share
             personal information.

Group Discussion:

I.   Are you a private person or do you like to talk about yourself?
     a. On a scale of 1 to 5 how talkative are you? 1= not at all
         talkative or 5= very talkative.
     b. People who are very talkative are more likely to share too
         much personal information with others.
II. What is personal information?
     a. information about your health
     b. information about your feelings
     c. information about your medication
     d. information about your placement in the hospital
     e. information about your problems
     f. *"Any others?"*
III. A therapy group setting is a confusing place because it seems
     like everyone knows about your private information. But even
     here you should not share all of your private information with
     everyone.
IV. Who should you share personal information with?
     a. DOCTOR – because they can't fully help you with
         medication and illnesses unless they have all of the
         information. Also, they are required by law to keep all of
         your information private because that is part of their job.
     b. POLICE – if you are ever questioned by the police it is
         important that you are honest and answer any questions
         they ask, but you can and should wait until someone you
         trust is there with you.
V.   Who can you share personal information with?
     a. CASE WORKER- if they are helping you with a job, your
         family, or a place to live they many need to know personal
         information to help get you the right things.
     b. STAFF – a person who is helping you with a problem or
         that you know very well.

       c. FAMILY
       d. FRIEND
  VI. Who should you not share personal information with?
       a. STRANGER
       b. SOMEONE YOU HAVE ONLY KNOWN A SHORT TIME
       c. SOMEONE AT YOUR PLACEMENT THAT YOU HAVEN'T MET
       d. SOMEONE YOU MEET IN THE COMMUNITY

Activity: Card Sort

Place icons of people or write the words on the board. Then provide different hypothetical pieces of personal information and have the residents sort the category of person they would share that information with. This can be done with each person individually, partners or as a group activity.

ICONS

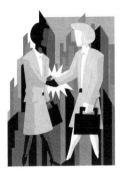 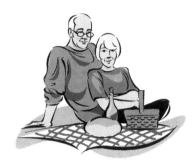

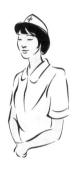 

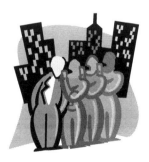 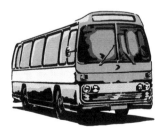

LEISURE SKILLS

Sessions: 1. Leisure Activities and Times to Enjoy Them

GOAL: The goal for this module is to assist residents in
              identifying things they enjoy so they can
              enjoy independent activities and time.

Leisure Activities and Times to Enjoy Them

Goal: To increase the person's independence and enjoyment of leisure time.

Objective: To be able to identify the several choices of things to do with free time and to include enjoyable activities in the person's daily schedules.

Group Discussion:

   I. What is **leisure time**?
- a. Free time spent doing something you enjoy.
- b. The time can be spent alone or with other people.
- c. This time should include relaxing and fun activities.
- d. "Any others?"

  II. Leisure Activities
- a. Arts and Crafts (drawing, painting)
- b. Sewing
- c. Watching movies
- d. Playing games with friends
- e. Reading
- f. Writing
- g. Sports
- h. Exercise
- i. Cooking
- j. Listening to music
- k. Dancing
- l. Yoga
- m. Bird watching
- n. Collecting things
- o. "Any others?"

 III. The purpose of leisure activities.
- a. to relax
- b. to enjoy yourself
- c. to socialize
- d. to structure time while you are waiting for something
- e. to take your mind off things that are upsetting
- f. "Any other reasons?"

 IV. Times to engage in leisure activities
- a. Free time
- b. When you are waiting for something
- c. When you are upset and need a break

      d. When you would like to calm down

      e. "Any other times?"

V.   One of the hardest things is remembering all of the choices you have when you are bored or looking for something to do. Having a picture list can be a great reminder.

Activity: My Favorite Things to Do

    Help residents make a list of their favorite things to do. Then help them make icons or pictures so that they can look at the list when they are bored or looking for something to do. It is usually difficult to remember all of the options, and the list is a great reminder.

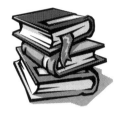 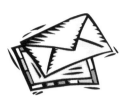 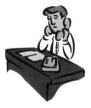 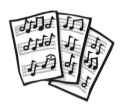

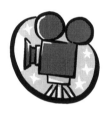 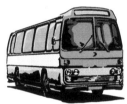 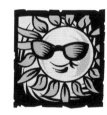 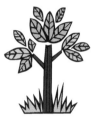

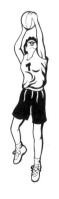 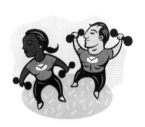 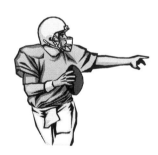

MONEY MANAGEMENT

Sessions: 1. Collecting and Monitoring Money
2. Spending and Monitoring Money

GOAL: The goal for this module is to assist residents in developing and maintaining the skills to collect, manage, and spend money with care and responsibility.

Collecting and Monitoring Money

Goal: To increase knowledge and understanding of their financial status and source of their money.

Objective: To be able to identify the source of their money, how much they receive monthly and where it is saved.

Group Discussion:

  I.   Where does your money come from?
       a.   Social Security
       b.   San Diego Regional Center
       c.   Work
       d.   Family
  II. Where does your money go when it comes?
       a.   bank
       b.   financial/business office
       c.   staff person
       d.   yourself
  III. How much money do you get?
  IV. How do you monitor how much money you have at a time?
       a.   ask a staff person or advocate
       b.   talk to your regional center case worker
  V.   What is a "Money Log"?
       a.   A book that keeps track of your money
            1.   how much you have
            2.   how much you get
            3.   how much you spend

Activity: Money Log

Help residents make their own money log. It would be great to include 5 to 10 minute appointments with someone from the business department to assist them in identifying how much they have.

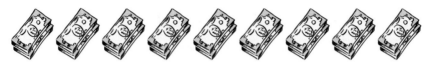

MONEY LOG

DATE	My money!	I earned. (added)	I spent. (took away)	What is left?
Sample: 9/5/11	$100	$50	XXX	$150
9/6/11	$150	XXX	$10	$140

Spending and Monitoring Money

Goal: To increase knowledge and understanding of their financial status and how to manage their money.

Objective: To be able to identify how much money they have and how to monitor their spending, including establishing a savings.

Group Discussion:

I. How do you know how much money you have?
   a. financial/business office
   b. regional center case manager
   c. money log
   d. staff person can help you find out?

II. What do you like to spend your money on? This is called *"FUN MONEY"*
   a. restaurants
   b. personal items
   c. candy
   d. cigarettes
   e. clothes
   f. outings

III. What do you need to spend your money on? This is called *"NEED MONEY"*
   a. clothes
   b. medication
   c. daily food
   d. appointments
   e. uniforms for work
   f. bills (phone, cable)

IV. What does it mean to budget your money?
   a. Each month you only have a limited amount of money you can spend.
   b. You will need to decide how that money is spent.
   c. This means saving for things that you may not "want" but you "need"
   d. This also means planning into the future.

V. How do you decide how to spend your money?
   a. First, decide how much money you *"NEED"*
   b. Second, decide how much you have left over for *"FUN MONEY"*

    c. Third, take out money you want to save.

VI. Savings Account!!!!

    a. After you take out money that you "need" for items such as clothes, food, bills, medication, etc.—How much do you have left over?

    b. Decide how much of the leftover money you want to put into a savings account.

    c. The same day every month (or when you receive your money) take out a set amount and put it aside into a savings account. That money will build up for when you need it or want something you don't have enough for each month.

Activity: **Sample Budget**

Help residents identify how much money they receive every month. A 5 to 10 minute appointment with a person from the financial or business office may be helpful for this. Then assist them in dividing the money into:

1. *"NEED MONEY"*
2. Savings
3. *"FUN MONEY"*

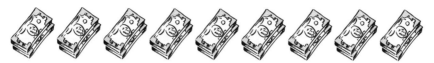

My Personal Budget

DATE	"NEED MONEY"	"WANT MONEY"	SAVINGS
SAMPLE 9/5/11	$75	$50	$25

Group Training and Activities

Topic: **SELF-CARE**

Sessions:
1. Hygiene - appearance
2. Hygiene – body odor (can be combined with session 1)
3. Privacy
4. Medication

GOAL: The goal for this module is to assist residents in developing and maintaining the skills to care for themselves in the most independent way they can so that they can lead dignified lives in a community setting.

Hygiene – Appearance

Goal: To present in a socially acceptable manner in the community to facilitate positive work and social interactions.

Objective: To identify a manner of appearance that is acceptable in the work place, social settings, and home.

Group Discussion:
I. What is included in physical appearance?
    a. Clothes
        1. Are they clean?
        2. Are they wrinkled?
        3. Do they smell nice?
        4. Do they show too much of the body?
    b. Hair
        1. Is it clean?
        2. Is it brushed?
        3. Is it covering the face and eyes?
    c. Clean skin
        1. Is it clean?
        2. Is make-up appropriate for women (too dark or smeared)?
        3. Are the men clean shaven or is their facial hair trimmed?
        4. Is there dirt under the fingernails?
    d. Teeth
        1. Are they brushed?
        2. Do they look clean?
        3. Is breath fresh?
II. Identify settings that physical appearance is considered.
    a. Work
    b. Community Outings
    c. Home
III. Why is physical appearance important?
     How might others act different toward you depending on how you look and smell?

Activity: Collage
Use magazines and newspapers to cut out pictures that represent appropriate and inappropriate work place

attire. Then cut out pictures for social gatherings, going to dinner or shopping, being home alone, and in public areas of the house.

Hygiene – Body Odor

Goal: To present in a socially acceptable manner in the community to facilitate positive work and social interactions.

Objective: To identify a routine of cleaning and areas of focus on the body vulnerable to body odor.

Group Discussion:
   I.   What is body odor?
  II.   How do you get body odor?
      a. Anyone can get body odor if they do not shower or bathe at least every other day.
      b. Body odor is worse if:
          1. a person sweats or is very active
          2. a person eats foods with a strong smell
          3. a person is wearing unclean clothes
          4. a person does not wear deodorant

 III. How do you prevent body odor?
      a. Take a shower or bath every day or at least every other day.
      b. Wash the parts of the body that are more likely to start to smell.
          1. underarms
          2. private parts
          3. feet
      c. Wear deodorant
 IV. How would you know if you have body odor?
      a. People say something to you
      b. You have not taken a shower or bath in two days
      c. People are avoiding standing near you
      d. Smell your clothes for the odor

Activity:

Ask residents about whether they notice other people's body odor and how important it is for them to smell nice. Assist residents in developing a hygiene kit that includes their favorite cleaning products. The kit can include a list or pictures from magazines and ads of products they wish to purchase. Put the list or pictures in a box. Possible products include:

Soap brand

Shampoo and conditioner brands

Shaving cream

Bath gels

Perfume or cologne

Lotion

Deodorant

Facial creams

Toothpaste

Privacy

Goal: To understand their own personal boundaries and know how to protect those boundaries.

Objective: To learn about their personal boundaries and sensitivities. Also, to know that it is *always* their choice whether or not they are touched and to learn what to do if someone violates those boundaries.

Group Discussion:

I. What are private parts?
    a. Both males and females have private parts of their bodies.
        - For men and boys those parts are the bottom and penis.
        - For women and girls those parts are the bottom, breasts, and vagina.

    Depending on the individual, it may be appropriate to use words that they have already learned. When making this decision, consider the age appropriateness of the word. For example, an adult should know the words suggested. Depending on the individual it may be most useful to first teach the person about his or her own body simply with the knowledge that men (boys) and women (girls) have different private parts.

    b. Private parts are to be kept covered when in public, that is why they are called "private." Remember, men (boys) and women have different private parts. That is why it is O.K. for men (boys) not to wear a shirt in public, but it not O.K. for women not to wear a shirt in public. That is also why we all wear swimming suits.

II. What are some times you may be asked to show our private parts to other people?
    a. One time would be when you go to the doctor. The doctor needs to check all parts of your body to make sure you are healthy.
    b. For individuals who need help bathing or dressing, another time is when someone is helping you change your clothes. Until you learn how to button your shirt, someone may need to help you.

    OR

    c. Someone needs to be in the bathroom when you take a shower to make sure you are safe or help you wash your body so that is another time when someone would need to see your private parts.

III. What are some ways you can protect your privacy?

    a. Always change clothes with the door closed or in a private place.

    b. Always wear a robe when you are leaving a shower or around other people.

    c. Keep your body covered when in public areas.

    d. Knock on any door that is closed before entering, even your own door if you have a roommate.

IV. What are some ways you can protect your body?

    a. If someone asks you to touch them in any way and you don't want to, you **never** have to.

    b. You are always in charge of who touches or sees your body.

    c. If you see someone without clothes on tell a staff person right away.

    d. If anyone ever asks you to show or touch the private parts of your or their body, the staff will always support you in protecting yourself.

Activity:

Help the residents identify ways they are focused on protecting their body (wearing a robe, changing clothes in private, telling others they don't want to be touched, etc.)

Help each resident identify at least one person they would tell if someone touched them or crossed their personal boundaries.

Medication

Goal: To understand the purpose of their medication and
            promote independence with medication management.

Objective: To identify the purpose of their medication, possible
            side effects, administration procedure, and who to talk
            to about changes or concerns.

Group Discussion:

  I.   What are some purposes for medication?
       a. Medical reasons (high blood pressure, diabetes, illness, etc.)
       b. Emotional reasons (depression, impulsivity, high energy, etc.)
  II. What are some ways medications are given?
       a. pill
       b. rub on skin
       c. shot
       d. inhaler
  III. What are some possible side effects?
       a. loss or increase in appetite
       b. sleepy
       c. headaches
       d. nausea
       e. feel jittery
  IV. What you need to know about your medication?
       a. What is the name of it?
       b. How much and how often to take it?
       c. What is it for?
       d. How might I feel on it?
       e. What are the side effects?
       f. What do I do if I don't like it?

Activity:

            Assist group members in filling out the attached personal
            medication chart. If the person does not read or write help
            them draw pictures whenever possible. For example, for
            dose the person can draw pictures of the number of pills
            taken and for time they can draw a picture of a clock the
            number of times they take it in a day (one, two or three
            clocks). All group members should draw a picture of the
            pill including shape and color in the last box.

My Medication Record

Medication Name	Dose	Times	Picture

WORK READINESS

Sessions: 1. Developing Work Readiness Skills
             2. Job Match
             3. Responsible Workplace Behavior

GOAL: The goal for this module is to assist residents in
             developing and maintaining the skills to be a desirable
             employee, socially appropriate, and an efficient worker.

Developing Work Readiness Skills

Goal: To develop the skills necessary to maintain a job of their choice.

Objective: To be able to identify goals and skills and behavior patterns needed to be an employable person.

Group Discussion:

   I. What is an employee?

   a. A person who is paid by a company or agency to complete a specific job.

   II. What makes a good employee or worker?

   a. Most important: Is always safe

   b. On time

   c. Dresses appropriately

   d. Works hard

   e. Is a good listener

   f. Is always polite

   III. What do you need to practice to **"Be Safe"**

   a. Communicate using words

   b. Keep your body from touching other people

   c. No hitting, kicking, biting, threatening, or hurting yourself.

   d. Communicating in SAFE and RESPECTFUL ways, even when you are angry or upset.

   IV. What do you need to practice to be **"On Time"**

   a. Set alarm or respond politely when someone wakes you up

   b. Get up early enough to allow for time to dress, eat, wash, brush teeth, and shave.

   c. Be at the pick-up spot five minutes early (bus stop, staff van, with staff)

   V. What do you need to practice to **"Dress Appropriate"**?

   a. Clothes should be clean and ironed.

   b. Body should be clean

   c. Clothes should cover all private areas of body.

   d. Clothes should include long pants (skirt for women is okay), shirts with sleeves and usually collars, and often closed toed shoes.

   e. Clothes should not have holes or stains.

   VI. What do you need to practice to **"Work Hard"**?

   a. Listen to the staff when they ask you to do something.

b. Try to do things on your own.

c. Practice sitting at a table working on a project for as long as you can without getting up.

d. Practice doing things you have never tried before.

VII. What do you need to practice being a **"Good Listener"**?

a. Make eye contact with staff when they are talking to you.

b. Listen to other people talk before you respond or say anything.

c. Follow directions when someone asks for your help.

VIII. What do you need to practice being **"Polite"**?

a. Tell people how you feel using a calm voice.

b. Be a **good listener.**

c. When you are angry communicate in a **safe** way.

d. Talk to staff about how to deal with problems that are frustrating.

e. Say "Please" and "Thank you" when talking to others.

f. Greet others with "Hi" and "How are you?"

Activity: "Work Clothes"

Gather a group of magazines with a lot of pictures of people. Have residents cut out pictures of people that they feel present with a nice look. It is important to include magazines of various styles (including inappropriate dress) for choice and discussion.

Job Match

Goal: To develop the skills necessary to maintain a job of their choice.

Objective: To be able to identify types of jobs that will be good fit with their skill set and personality style.

Group Discussion:

I.   What type of jobs do you think look fun or interesting?

II. Job Match Profile

  a. What type of things do you like to do?
      1. arts and crafts
      2. build things
      3. talk to people
      4. clean
      5. yard work
      6. work with money
      7. help people
      8. fix things

  b. What things are you good at?
      1. working with your hands
      2. building things
      3. counting
      4. interacting with others
      5. organizing
      6. doing things fast

  c. What are some things about you that are important to know when choosing a job?
      1. What is your sleep schedule?
      2. What time of day do you like to work hard?
      3. Do you like to work alone or with others?
      4. Do you like to be sitting or active when you are working?
      5. Do you like to work inside or outside?

III. What things do you think you need to learn to get the job you want?

    How do you learn those things?

  a. There may be job that you don't love, but that will teach you things you need to learn to get a better job.

  b. It may be more important to earn money for awhile at an okay job at the same time you are looking for a better one.

Activity: Job Match Profile

Help residents complete a job match profile.

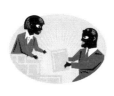 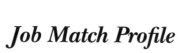 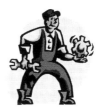

Job Match Profile

1. WHAT TYPE OF THINGS DO YOU LIKE TO DO?

    A.

    B.

    C.

2. WHAT THINGS ARE YOU GOOD AT?

    A.

    B.

    C.

3.   WHAT ARE SOME THINGS ABOUT YOU THAT ARE IMPORTANT TO KNOW WHEN CHOOSING A JOB?

A.

B.

C.

"So, I would like a job that I can _____ or _____

and I would like to work with people who are _____

and _____.

It is important that my job is not _____.

Responsible Workplace Behavior

Goal: To develop the skills necessary to maintain a job of their choice.

Objective: To be able to practice and utilize appropriate behavior for a workplace, including responsible work habits and appropriate social interactions.

Group Discussion:

I.   Describe a great employee or worker?
   a.   Hard worker
   b.   Dependable
   c.   Polite and Respectful
II.   What do you do to be a **Hard Worker?**
   a.   Try your best every day.
   b.   When you are bored or tired you complete your work anyway.
   c.   You try new things.
   d.   You follow instructions.
   e.   You try to work on your own, but ask questions any time something is confusing.
III.   What do you do to be dependable?
   a.   You are on time every day.
   b.   You call your boss if you are going to be late or miss a day.
   c.   You listen to instructions and ask questions any time you are confused.
IV.   What do you do to be **Polite and Respectful**?
   a.   You talk in a quiet tone of voice.
   b.   You listen to your boss, giving eye contact and letting them know you understand.
   c.   You go to work with a smile and say "hi" to your co-workers.
   d.   You say "Please" when you are asking someone for something.
   e.   You say "Thank you" when someone has done something for you or said something nice about you.
   f.   You use polite language, no swearing or teasing others.
V.   It is also important that you do not deal with any personal problems at work.
   a.   If you are upset with someone in your private life or home, you do not discuss it at work.

    b. If you are angry with a staff member, you do not discuss it at work.

    c. If you are frustrated with something or someone at work, you can ask for a meeting with your boss and discuss it there.

    d. When you are at work, you are there to complete a job only.

VI. It is very important that you are PROFESSIONAL.

    a. Wear appropriate clothing

    b. Deal with problems as the responsible adult that you are.

    c. Treat others with dignity and respect

    d. Act with dignity and respect.

Activity: Set Goals

Help residents identify what areas they already have great skills. Praise and point out good examples of positive behavior patterns and how it can relate to the work place. Then help each resident identify one (or two) areas that they would like help to improve. Identify options for them to work on the goals and how staff can help them. This should then be communicated to line staff so everyone can help them.

Role Play

Here are some examples of role-play scenarios that are common for our individuals in a work setting:

1. If you are feeling tired or bored at work, what do you do?

   Let's practice...sit at the table and think about being tired and bored. What do you do?

2. If you are angry about not being able to smoke a cigarette when you want, what do you do?

   Let's practice...ask a staff if you can take a break and smoke a cigarette. The staff says "No", what do you do?

3. If you think someone at work is cute, what do you do about it? What if it is an employee?

   Let's practice...you are sitting at the table and the man/woman you think is cute walks by, what do you do?

4. You show up late for work because you were having a hard time in the morning, how do you apologize?

   Let's practice...You walk into the office and you are 15 minutes late...what do you say?

5. If someone is teasing you, what do you do?

   Let's practice...you are working at a table and someone walks by and laughs at your shoes...what do you do or say?

6. You are unhappy with the job you are being asked to do, what do you do?

   Your boss just asked you to continue folding envelopes, which you have been doing all morning and don't want to do anymore... what do you do or say?

Transitional Planning Information and Preparation Form

NAME: _____

AGE: _____

CURRENT RESIDENCE: _____

DIAGNOSES: _____

_____

_____

PLACEMENT HISTORY

1. What were the individual's previous living arrangements? This should include the type of living arrangements and the length of time the individual resided in each place.

2. Were any of the living arrangements successful for the individual? Which arrangements worked best and why did the person have to leave?

3. Which living arrangements were unsuccessful? What happened and why didn't they work?

4. If the individual has the verbal skills, can he or she identify a preferred living situation? If this arrangement is not feasible due to the person's medical and/or behavioral challenges, what would it take to help the person reach the goal?

5. If the person is currently residing in an institution, how long has it been since the individual lived in the community? If the individual is not ready to move to the community, what skills or types of supports are needed in order to support a discharge from the institution?

6. If living in an institutionalized setting, has the person ever had to change units or residences within the facility? Was the change the result of the individual's behaviors or medical needs and how did the person adjust to the change? Did the change result in an increase in behavioral challenges or an increase in psychiatric symptoms?

7. Does the individual's family support a move to the community and to a less structured setting? If not what are the family's concerns?

8. Does the individual have a history of psychiatric hospitalizations? If so, how frequent were the hospitalizations and what prompted the admissions?

DEVELOPMENTAL HISTORY

1. What is the cause of the individual's intellectual disability? Is a syndrome involved? If so, does that syndrome have behavioral or medical symptoms that need to be considered in placement planning?

2. Does the person have a diagnosis in the autistic spectrum that has implications for the type of living arrangements and environmental surroundings?

COMMUNICATION ABILITIES

1. What is the extent of the individual's expressive language? How does the person currently communicate wants, needs, preferences, dislikes, etc? Is it through purposeful reach, pointing, or verbally?

2. Does the individual use any augmentative communication device or any communication system that would require training for future care providers?

3. Does the person have any hearing deficits that impact communicative abilities?

4. Does the person use American Sign Language (ASL) or unique manual signs?

5. What is the individual's receptive language skill level? Can the person understand basic verbal instructions and do instructions and questions need to be presented in a certain way? For example, should communications be provided by care providers using concrete, short sentences with no more than one-step instructions provided at any given time?

6. Does the individual exhibit episodes of prolonged or loud vocalizations that could be disruptive to others in the home or the neighbors?

7. How does the individual communicate when in pain?

SOCIAL RELATIONSHIPS

1. Does the person enjoy being alone? How social is the person?

2. Does the individual enjoy spending time with care providers and/or peers?

3. Who is included in and what is the extent of the person's current support system?

4. What kind of peer group does the individual need?

5. Does the person respond better to male or female care providers?

6. Does the person want to leave his or her current social support system?

7. Is the family in contact with the individual? If so, to what degree are they in contact and are those relationships conflictual?

8. To what extent does the person need assistance from care providers to facilitate social relationships?

LIKES AND DISLIKES

1. What are the individual's likes and dislikes?

2. What kind of community activities does the person enjoy?

3. Currently, what is the frequency with which the person accesses activities in the community?

4. Does the person exhibit any behavioral challenges while in the community that may require enhanced supervision?

5. What kind of leisure skills and hobbies does the person have? What does the person enjoy doing with his or her free time?

6. Does the individual need the support of care providers to engage in these hobbies or leisure activities?

7. Does the person need a very active daily schedule or does the person prefer to be more sedentary?

SELF-HELP SKILLS

Toileting

1. With regard to toileting, is the individual continent? What level of assistance does the person need with toileting needs?

2. Does the person have issues with constipation that require such interventions as the administration of a suppository? If so, would this require a certain level of nursing care in the residence?

3. Is there a history of nighttime incontinence that would require a care provider to assist the individual during the night?

4. Does the person exhibit any behavioral challenges around toileting that would require enhanced care provider supervision, such as smearing feces, compulsively flushing the toilet, or flooding the bathroom by turning on the faucets, etc.?

Grooming/bathing/dressing

1. With regard to grooming, bathing, and dressing, what level of assistance does the person require from care providers (e.g., verbal prompts, hand-over-hand assistance, total care, etc.)?

2. How cooperative is the individual in performing self-care tasks? If care provider assistance is needed, does the person refuse assistance or become combative? Is self-care assistance going to be potentially time consuming for a care provider?

3. Does the person have a seizure disorder which would require monitoring while showering to ensure safety?

4. Does the individual need adaptive equipment for any of the self-care tasks such as a pedestal bath, etc.?

5. Does the person display any tactile defensiveness which increases resistiveness when care providers try to assist?

6. What is the individual's current schedule or routine with regard to these activities? For example, does the person prefer to take a shower in the morning or evening? Is it important to maintain the current routine?

7. Are there any clothing preferences? For example, does the person dislike wearing shoes with laces?

8. Are there any compulsive or ritualistic behaviors exhibited by the individual around any of the self-care tasks that interfere with the completion of the tasks?

Eating

1. What level of assistance is required around eating? Is the individual independent with eating?

2. Does the person have any unsafe eating habits such as eating too quickly, taking bites that are too big, or stealing food? Would any of these unsafe eating habits pose a health and safety risk to the individual if not carefully monitored? Does the person require enhanced supervision during mealtimes? Does the individual have any choking risks due to unsafe eating habits or due to dysphagia that would required special diets and/or special monitoring? Do any facility modifications need to be made to the residence or facility prior to the individual moving in?

3. Have there been any issues around food that have been problematic for the individual, such as compulsively drinking water (i.e., psychogenic polydypsia) or an eating disorder?

MEDICAL CONSIDERATIONS

1. What are the individual's current medical conditions and does the person require specialized care such as nursing services?

2. Are the conditions currently symptomatic or asymptomatic and what level of monitoring is required?

3. Are there any medical conditions which are progressive? Is the person's health status likely to deteriorate in the near future? If so, would the individual's health care needs exceed the living arrangement currently being considered?

4. Have there been any recent hospitalizations? If so, is the person medically stable enough to consider a move?

5. When the individual has been ill, is there a history of quickly succumbing to the illness with a slow recovery?

6. Does the person have any current medical conditions that may be exacerbated by the stress of a move? For example, does the individual have high blood pressure or any cardiac issues that may be impacted by stress? Does this require special monitoring or follow-up?

7. Are there any medical conditions that are considered restricted health care conditions in the community and require specific health care plans that need to be reviewed by a local licensing agency?

8. Does the individual have any conditions that can be contagious to others, such as a form of hepatitis? Are there additional vaccinations required for the people working with the individual?

9. If the individual moves to the community, how readily available are the community medical resources and supports? Is gaining access to these supports going to be difficult?

10. Are there any past medical conditions that may re-occur? If so, what were the signs and symptoms exhibited by the individual when ill? What treatments were provided and were they effective?

11. Does the individual have a seizure disorder? How well controlled are the seizures and what types of interventions have been needed? For example, does oxygen need to be available or has the individual required injections in response to multiple seizures?

12. With regard to motor skills, is the person able to walk independently? Does the person need assistance from others and what degree of assistance is needed?

13. Does the individual have an unsteady gait which increases the likelihood of falls?

14. Does the individual have any visual impairments, and if so, what is the extent of the vision difficulties? Does this require any environmental modifications?

15. Are there any sensory integration issues that require environmental modifications?

16. Does the individual require any special dietary modifications or nutritional supports?

BEHAVIORAL CHALLENGES

1. What are the individual's current behavioral challenges? How frequently do they occur and how severe are they?

2. Are there identifiable antecedents or precursors?

3. Are there any restrictive interventions or devices being used to address the behaviors that would not be allowed in a community facility due to licensing regulations? This would include various forms of restraints such as wrist-to-waist restraints, helmets, etc. Can the use of these devices be faded out or discontinued prior to the individual leaving an institutionalized setting?

4. What are the histories of these behaviors? How long have they been occurring?

5. Are there any "behavioral alerts" (i.e., challenging behaviors that have not been identified as specific target behaviors, since they do not occur with sufficient intensity or severity to warrant an intervention)? These would include any behaviors that staff working in an institution encounter on a day-to-day basis or encounter so frequently that they take them for granted. However, these behaviors in a less structured or less restrictive setting, such as the community, may pose a problem.

6. Do any of the behavioral challenges impact participation in community outings or attendance at a day program?

7. Since old behavioral challenges can resurface under stress, what is the history of the behavioral challenges?

8. How does the person respond to change? Does it increase the frequencies or severities of the behavioral challenges?

9. What interventions, both proactive and reactive strategies, have been used to address the behavioral challenges?

10. Does the person have a psychiatric diagnosis? How are the symptoms of the psychiatric condition being addressed? Is the psychiatric condition being considered in creating the treatment goals or in creating any of the behavioral intervention plans?

11. Does the person currently suffer from insomnia or have a history of insomnia that may reoccur with the stress of a move? What level of staffing or supervision does this require?

12. If the person is aggressive, how frequent are the episodes of aggression and how intense are the incidents? Have they resulted in any injuries to the person or to others? What level of staffing is needed to intervene and de-escalate the behaviors?

13. Does the individual have a trauma history and, if so, in what type of environment did the trauma occur? What type of trauma was it (e.g., sexual abuse, physical abuse)?

Appendix E

Sample Behavior Data Form

This is a sample behavior data form that was developed for a group home that was having difficulty keeping consistent data. It was developed with the input of the staff and found to be very effective in gathering the appropriate data. In addition, the staff completed it more consistently than any other data system before this one. It does not include all of the detailed information that the clinical team wanted, but the staff felt comfortable with this form. As discussed in this book, it is more important to have consistent data collection than to have the perfect data collection system. If the staff are not consistently completing the forms, the data is not useful and can be misleading. This form allowed for consistent data collection across many group homes and a large staff group.

House Name
CLIENT BEHAVIOR DATA FORM

NAME: **DATE:** _____   **Staff Initials**_____

TIME OF DAY	Leisure and Community Integration	Aggression a. attempt b. physical c. verbal	Property Destruction a. <$5 b. $5-$20 c. >$20	Calling 911 a. attempt b. success
7 am				
8 am				
9 am				
10 am				
11 am				
12 pm				
1 pm				
2 pm				
3 pm				
4 pm				
5 pm				
6 pm				
7 pm				
8 pm				
Overnight				

* Complete Functional Analysis on reverse side for any behaviors displayed.

Did you have today any of the following concerns or observations? (Please include details in narrative form in observation and functional analysis part below)

	Health concerns: Note any changes in physical condition, as well as signs of illnesses or injuries.		Changes in sleep - patterns: Unusual sleep pattern (Awake at night, asleep during the day)		Day program or school reports, visits, telephone conversations, mail, concerns.		Family contacts: Visits (on or off site), concerns, mail, phone conversations, etc.		Mood changes: Unusual crying, withdrawal, anxiety, anger, etc.	
	Yes	No	Yes	No	Yes	No	Yes	No	Yes	No
AM										
PM										
ON										

FUNCTIONAL ANALYSIS AND DAILY OBSERVATIONS

1) Time	Describe what you observed before a behavior, the behavior itself, and what you observed afterwards. Record all observations (not only observations of problematic and disruptive behaviors), such as new skills learned, pro-social behavior, pleasurable experiences, preferred and non-preferred activities, etc. Include any health concerns, family visits, school or day program concerns, changes in sleep and mood patterns. Note if an SIR was written.	2) Staff Initials

Index

processing 18, 173
profile 16, 47, 57, 103, 117, 152, 160, 236
compulsions 33-35
Compulsive Behavior Checklist 35
concentration 18, 26, 27
confusion 10, 13, 26, 48, 104, 134
coping skills 20-21, 110, 117, 120, 134

D

data
  baseline 87, 99-100
  collection 70, 98-101, 104, 257
  duration recording 100-101
  frequency/event recording 100-101
  interval recording 100-101
  narrative recording 100
  scatter plots 101
  system 2, 9, 44, 64, 70, 78, 85, 101-102, 104, 116, 119, 124-126, 142, 144, 157, 163, 168, 184, 194, 245-247, 257
  time sampling 101
Delusional Disorder 39
Dementia 54
Dependent Personality Disorder 45, 48
depression 25, 27, 91
developmental disorders 2, 145, 152, 174, 184
developmental history 74
developmental milestones 13, 74
developmental shift 13
direct care staff. See care providers
discharge planning 121, 139
disorganized speech 37
distractibility 30
DM-ID 23, 25, 29, 37, 44, 50, 95, 157-160
D-N-A 106
DSM-IV-TR
  Adjustment Disorder 37
  Antisocial Personality Disorder 44, 47, 164
  Attention Deficit Hyperactivity Disorder (ADHD) 87
  Avoidant Personality Disorder 45, 48
  Bipolar Disorder 28, 30, 50, 77

Borderline Personality Disorder (BPD) 46
Brief Psychotic Disorder 39
Delusional Disorder 39
Dependent Personality Disorder 45, 48
Due to a General Medical Condition 30, 50
Dysthymia 25
Generalized Anxiety Disorder (GAD) 31
Histrionic Personality Disorder 45-47
Intermittent Explosive Disorder 49, 50, 77, 164, 165
Major Depression 25
Narcissistic Personality Disorder 45-47
Obsessive-Compulsive Disorder (OCD) 34, 48, 50, 82, 148, 150
Obsessive-Compulsive Personality Disorder (OCPD) 48
Panic Disorder 32
Paranoid Personality Disorder 44-45
Personality Disorder, Not Otherwise Specified 44, 49
Posttraumatic Stress Disorder (PTSD) 35
Schizoaffective Disorder 39, 40, 77
Schizoid Personality Disorder 44-45
Schizophrenia 37-39, 50, 91, 150-151, 163
Schizophreniform Disorder 38
Schizotypal Personality Disorder 44-45
  with psychotic features 40
Dual Diagnosis 1
Due to a General Medical Condition 30, 50
Dysthymia 25

E

elevated mood 29
emotional considerations 13
endocrine 43, 52
executive functioning 16, 20-21, 51, 110, 119, 142

F

fatigue   10, 18, 25, 53, 63, 65, 93-94, 103, 151, 172
flat affect   37, 45
Fragile X Syndrome   65, 74
functional analysis   98, 258

G

gastrointestinal conditions
  constipation   61-62, 83, 127, 154-155, 249
  dysphagia   60
  gastroesophageal reflux   53, 61-62, 157
general medical condition   30-31, 50, 262
Generalized Anxiety Disorder (GAD)   31
generalized seizures   64

H

hallucination   43
head injury   74-75, 123
hedonistic activities.   30
Histrionic Personality Disorder   45-47
hopelessness   24
hygiene   196, 224-225, 227
hyperactivity   50, 71, 87, 90, 164
hypersomnia   25
hyperthyroidism   65
hypomanic   28, 30, 87
hypothesis   70, 102, 105

I

Impulse Control Disorders   49
initial planning team conferences   133
insomnia   25, 53-54, 132, 148, 256
intellectual disability
  mild   6, 13, 31, 37, 45, 52, 61, 94, 158
  moderate   6, 13, 37, 40, 62, 94, 193
  profound   4-5, 11, 26, 28, 40, 45, 71, 89, 165
  severe   2, 4-5, 11, 26, 28, 33, 40, 45, 50, 52-53, 61-63, 70-71, 80, 89, 131, 158, 163, 165, 169, 178, 181, 193, 254
Intermittent Explosive Disorder   49, 50, 77, 164, 165

irritability   25-26, 28-31, 36-37, 47, 49, 63, 85, 163

L

language
  expressive   4, 7, 16-17, 26, 28-29, 40, 78, 88, 124, 133, 172, 245
  non-verbal   17, 20, 32, 34, 42, 59, 76, 78, 88-89, 118, 148, 165, 177
  receptive   16-18, 78, 125, 142, 152, 172, 246
law enforcement   1
leisure skills   87-88, 112
lethargy   11
long-term retrieval   16, 20, 110
low motivation   24

M

Major Depression   25
mania   28-30, 40
medical condition(s)
  cancer   62, 65
  cardiovascular   30
  circadian rhythm disorder   54
  endocrine   43, 52
  general medical condition   30-31, 50, 262
  hyperthyroidism   65
  metabolic   31, 43, 55
  nocturnal angina   32
  respiratory   30, 60, 63
  seizures   43, 50, 60, 64, 66, 130, 133, 151, 253
    generalized seizures   64
    partial seizures   43, 64
    Pseudoseizures   64
  sleep apnea   32, 53-54, 63, 66, 94, 95, 150-151, 153
  urological conditions   62
medical providers   4-5, 12, 67
medication
  psychotropic   53, 61-63, 69-71, 75-76, 83, 90, 94, 134, 139, 148, 172
  side effects   5, 10, 11, 18, 36, 54, 61, 63, 69, 70-72, 75-76, 94, 103, 138, 151, 166, 231
  target symptom approach   72

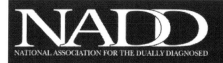

NADD
NATIONAL ASSOCIATION FOR THE DUALLY DIAGNOSED

132 Fair St., Kingston, NY 12401-4802
Phone (845) 331-4336 • (800) 331-5362
Fax (845) 331-4569
e-mail: info@thenadd.org
www.thenadd.org

Join NADD today!

It's easy to sign up:
Just go to **www.thenadd.org**

Membership Matters and You Make a Difference!

Members are an integral part of what makes the National Association for the Dually Diagnosed (NADD) a leader in the dissemination of state-of-the-art information. When joining NADD you will immediately be recognized as an individual who is concerned about the issues facing mental health care for persons who have intellectual disabilities. Simply by joining NADD you will become a prestigious member and have a voice in NADD's growing influential organization.

We invite you to join NADD today and build knowledge.

NADD is the leading organization providing professionals, educators, policy makers and families with education, training and information on mental health issues relating to persons with intellectual disabilities.

Education is important and NADD provides members with opportunity to learn more:

- Regional Conferences
- Annual Conferences
- International Conferences
- Teleconference Training
- Online Training (Continuing Education Credits)
- Onsite Consulting/Training for Government/Private Organizations

NADD Members receive discounts on all services and products

Over >>

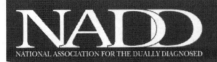
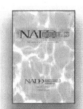
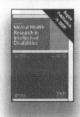
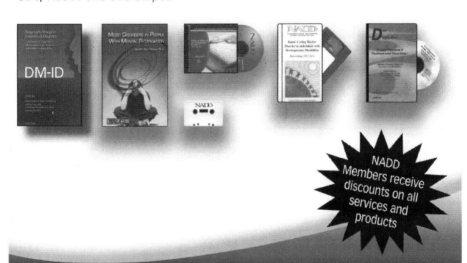